1990

SERVICE EXCELLENCE IN HEALTH CARE THROUGH THE USE OF COMPUTERS

AMERICAN COLLEGE OF HEALTHCARE EXECUTIVES MANAGEMENT SERIES

Anthony R. Kovner, Series Editor

Roger Kropf

Service Excellence in Health Care through the Use of Computers

MANAGEMENT SERIES
American College of Healthcare Executives

95 94 93 92 91 90   5 4 3 2 1

Library of Congress Cataloging-in-Publication Data

Kropf, Roger.
    Service excellence in health care through the use of computers / Roger Kropf.
    p.   cm. (Management series / American College of Healthcare Executives)
    Includes index.
    ISBN 0-910701-56-3 (hardbound)
    1. Health facilities—Administration—Data processing. 2. Medical care—Data processing. I. Title. II. Series.
    [DNLM 1. Computers. 2. Health Services—organization & administration 3. Information Systems. W 26.5 K93s]
RA971.6.K75   1990   362.1'1'068—dc20
DNLM/DLC for Library of Congress   90-4852 CIP

Health Administration Press
A division of the Foundation of the
  American College of Healthcare Executives
1021 East Huron Street
Ann Arbor, Michigan 48104-9990
(313) 764-1380

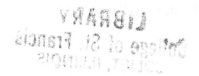

To Marcia, Andrew, and Sara—
who made it possible to get to the end.

Contents

Acknowledgments

This book could not have been written without the help of many people who shared with me their ideas about how information systems, strategic planning, and marketing all relate to each other. Carol Surprenant at the University of Rhode Island introduced me to the field of services marketing. Ted Stohr at New York University invited me to seminars' where I first learned about the concept of strategic information systems. Ken Bopp at the University of Missouri provided an invaluable framework for organizing the first part of this book in his articles on consumer satisfaction with health services.

A number of people helped to improve my understanding of how computer technology can improve service quality. Alex Szafran at Siemens Medical helped me think through the implications of teleradiology for the management of health services. John Nunnelly at HBO & Company and Janet Guptill at the Sachs Group explained how market analysis software could help plan services. Pam Hanlon at Integrated Medical Systems helped me understand the complexities of hospital-to-physician computer networks. Patsy Marr at New York University Medical Center contributed greatly to my understanding of the potential of hospital information services to serve nurses and physicians. Steve Duck at HealthLink provided critical information on how referral systems operate.

While many people helped in the preparation of the cases at the end of the book, I owe special thanks to Chuck Emery, Jr., at Samaritan Health Services, Judy Lester at the Cleveland Clinic, Marshall de G. Ruffin, Jr., at Inter+Net Health Systems, and Rich Colesanti at Vassar Brothers Hospital.

A number of people reacted to drafts and helped me improve the quality of this book. Tony Kovner at New York University provided his usual quick and incisive comments. Steve Tucker at Trinity University and Phil Reeves at

George Washington University helped sharpen my thinking about how to reach my intended audience. Barry Eisenberg at Sibley Memorial Hospital helped me to write in a way that would benefit experienced planning and marketing professionals.

Finally, I want to thank the many students in my information systems and planning and marketing courses whose questions made me better organize my thoughts on how these subjects could be related.

Preface

Employees, for the most part, want to do a good job; they want to give good service to their customers. If they're not doing it, more than likely something is standing in their way, and more than likely it's the organization. It's up to management to create the conditions that make service excellence possible and worthwhile. Employees will come through.

—Karl Albrecht, *At America's Service*

To succeed with service excellence in the long run, management has to establish support systems that give employees the power to serve the customer.

—Wendy Leebov, *Service Excellence*

This book is aimed at managers in health service organizations who, having heard the call for "service excellence" voiced by Tom Peters, Robert Waterman, Michael Porter, and other authors, are interested in finding out how that can be achieved in their organizations. Clearly, the selection and motivation of competent professionals is of paramount importance. Many of them hear on a daily basis, however, that the "systems don't work." This book is an attempt to outline how some systems could be made to work better—especially those which involve communications with the physician and the patient.

This book describes computer technologies that can improve the systems we use to provide health care—and increase patient and physician satisfaction. A range of such computer technologies are on the market. Examples are hardware and software for linking the physician's office to a hospital's information system, and systems that match patients to physicians and services that meet their preferences for location, hours of service, and other provider characteristics.

The major objective of this book is to inform managers of technologies that have the potential to improve services, and to stimulate their thinking about the role such technologies could play in achieving excellence in the delivery of health services. Special emphasis will be given to computer technologies that reach out to patients and physicians living and working beyond the walls of the organization. Such systems are less widely known and used in health care organizations.

Most of the technologies described in this book cost less than $100,000 to purchase. Few hospitals will, therefore, be in a position to automatically reject the idea of acquiring any of these technologies because of the cost, particularly when the benefits to physicians and patients are considered. A large hospital or multihospital system that implements several of the technologies to serve a large population could spend several million dollars, however. The major issue which this book will help managers resolve is how much to invest—and in what technologies.

Additional information on specific products will still have to be collected. This book is not a buyer's guide. It does not provide information on all the products on the market and evaluate them individually or in comparison with each other. In the time it takes for a book like this to be produced, such information would become outdated and inaccurate.

Two basic premises of this book are that creativity in the use of technology is critically important, and that health care managers need to learn from each other. For these reasons, a number of case studies of organizations that have used technology to improve service quality are provided.

The case studies also suggest that implementation will not be as easy as removing equipment from a carton and plugging it in. The technology provides a way for an organization to deliver a service. Delivering a level of service that is consistently excellent requires careful planning, continuous evaluation of performance, and the willingness to change. The alternative is remaining at, or regressing to, mediocrity.

Part I

Service Excellence and Computer Technology

1.

Introduction

Purpose of This Book

This book discusses how computer technology can be used to increase physician and patient satisfaction and lead to the excellence in the delivery of services discussed by Tom Peters and Robert Waterman, Jr., in *In Search of Excellence,*[1] and by Karl Albrecht and Ron Zemke in *Service America!*[2] By improving the value of services received, the use of computer technology could also lead to the type of sustainable competitive advantage described by Michael Porter in *Competitive Advantage.*[3] Porter's concepts of value analysis and his framework for understanding how sustainable competitive advantages are achieved are used in Chapter 3 to help managers select and implement a competitive strategy that includes the use of computer technology.

This book has four major purposes:

— To inform managers of computer technologies that could improve physician and patient satisfaction with health care services

— To stimulate thinking about new ways to use computer technologies

— To help in selecting a desirable array of computer technologies

— To suggest ways to improve the chances of successful implementation

The Technologies Described

Most of the technologies described in this book cost less than $100,000 to purchase. A few would cost more than a million dollars if implemented by a large hospital or multihospital system to serve a large population. Although many health care organizations may not be interested in a major investment, the benefits and relatively low cost of some of the technologies described make it important that managers be aware of their existence.

The technologies described in this book are:

— service referral and outbound telemarketing systems
— scheduling and tracking systems
— market analysis systems
— teleradiology
— technologies for communicating between providers, including computer links and fax

In selecting technologies for examination in this book, special emphasis was given to computer technologies that reach out to patients and physicians living and working beyond the walls of the organization. Such systems are less widely known and used in health care organizations.

Some technologies that could improve patient and physician satisfaction with services are not discussed because they are widely used in health care organizations and have been described in detail by other authors. They include order entry and results reporting systems, inventory and materials management systems, and billing systems. Managers who are interested in understanding the capabilities of such systems should consult books by Charles Austin,[4] Richard Sneider,[5] and Howard and Beatrice Rowland.[6]

Technologies in development have also not been described. This includes "smart cards," which can store medical records and other information on a plastic card the size of a credit card. The card contains either a computer memory chip (the same device that stores information in a personal computer) or uses a laser to burn the information on a piece of plastic (the way music is stored on a compact disk). Problems in the low-cost manufacture of such smart cards have delayed their use by American credit card companies, which in turn has made them expensive for smaller buyers like health insurance companies and hospitals.[7] No health care organization in the United States is known to be using them in routine operations at this time.

Achieving Service Excellence

Quality—The New Challenge in Health Care

Low hospital occupancies and lower than expected patient volume have put pressure on many hospitals, physicians, and other providers to increase volume. At the same time, books and articles have appeared on the poor quality of service offered by American companies and how to fix the problem. Some hospitals, physicians, and health care organizations have realized that "service excellence" may be the solution to low patient volume and declining market share. It may also be necessary to hold on to physicians and patients who believe that excellent service is their right.

At the same time, government, employers, and insurance companies are asking for proof that hospitals, physicians, and other health care providers provide high-quality services.

Making Improvements in Service Quality

This book will not focus on how standards defined by medical professionals for the structure, process, and outcomes of medical care can be achieved, that is, clinical quality. It will focus on how services are evaluated by patients and referring physicians, who often have limited knowledge of the standards used to evaluate clinical quality. They evaluate what will be called "service quality."

Patient evaluation

Patients evaluate a medical service by comparing the service they perceived they received with the service they expected. Patients are satisfied when the perceived service is equal to or better than they expected.[8]

Although patients seek medical services in order to improve their well-being, they have a limited ability to evaluate what Avedis Donabedian[9] calls the structure and process of care, and they cannot assess whether the outcome that is achieved is more or less favorable than what was possible. Patients therefore rely on their interpersonal interactions with staff and professionals, the assessment of friends and others they trust, and what they can see of the physical features of the service process (for example, the attractiveness of the facility and the newness of the equipment) in setting their initial expectations and in subsequent evaluations.

The focus of this book will be on those factors that affect patient perceptions of staff and physician:

— Caring (warm, interested, concerned, understanding, not dominating or talking down to the patient)

— Professionalism (congenial, accessible, conscientious, proficient, of high integrity)

— Competence (knowledgeable, efficient, capable, thorough)

Kenneth Bopp refers to these as "expressive caring," "expressive professionalism," and "expressive competence" to underscore that we are dealing with perceptions—what the consumer believes—and that those perceptions are based on what is expressed verbally and nonverbally in the encounter with staff, physicians, and other professionals.[10]

Referring physician evaluation

The factors that affect physician use of services are complex since the physician is capable of evaluating, to varying degrees, the clinical quality of the service. The focus of this book will be on factors that affect the *referring* physician's perceptions of:

— individualized patient management and care

— convenience to patient

— the degree to which patient preferences are met

— the frequency and completeness of communications received

— support for the practice, including reciprocations received

Although other factors determine referral behavior,[11] these are the ones that are most likely to be affected by the exchange of information.

Importance of having a strategy

Excellence in delivering services requires a strategy. Although experts differ, the following steps are often included:[12]

— Target a market.

— Succinctly describe the service you want to offer and the benefits it will provide to the target market.

— Make service excellence the primary goal of the organization.

— Create an organizational structure and systems that reinforce the importance of service excellence and support the front-line people providing services.

A strategy is needed to move beyond mediocre service because it forces the organization to make choices as to who the customer is, what benefits they are supposed to receive, and how the organization will deliver those benefits consistently over a sustained period of time.

Importance of changing staff behavior

The attitudes and behavior of staff are of major importance. Consumer perceptions of staff caring, professionalism, and competence are important factors in how consumers evaluate health services. Also, services are not created and then consumed later, like packaged goods. A quality check cannot be instituted after manufacture and before consumption. Consistently excellent delivery of services requires that staff act in a caring, professional, and competent manner consistently, often without a supervisor observing the process.

Considerable emphasis is therefore placed in the books and articles on service excellence on the importance of training, motivating, and supporting the front-line staff who provide services. In health care, this means everyone from nurses and physicians to receptionists and housekeeping staff.[13,14,15]

Importance of changing systems

Good people using bad systems do not usually produce excellent service over a long period of time. A scheduling system that will not let an office manager "fit in" a patient who wants to see the doctor, a lab information system that deletes tests after seven days although outpatients often see their physicians ten or more days after a test, a phone system that is always busy—all these can prevent the most motivated staff members from delivering excellent service.

Computer systems can play a role in supporting staff who want to deliver excellent service. They will not make disinterested staff provide adequate service or rationalize procedures that reduce efficiency. They are a tool, but often they can provide the difference between mediocre and excellent service.

Using Computer Technology to Improve Service Quality

A basic premise of this book is that computer technologies can play a major role in providing consistently excellent service to one or more targeted markets. Tables 1.1 and 1.2 summarize the potential benefits to patients and referring physicians of the use of the technologies described below.

Improving the Process

Health care involves some complex processes that provide many opportunities for improvement. Some techniques for identifying those opportunities are presented in this book. Examples of how computer technologies could help at several points in the process are described below.

Scheduling services

The computers of physicians, hospitals, and other organizations can be linked. Such computer links can improve the speed of scheduling by bypassing busy telephone systems and increase accuracy by replacing verbal requests and illegible notes with typed computer input.

Table 1.1   Potential Benefits to Patients of Selected Computer Technologies

| Technology | Enhanced Perception of | | |
	Caring	*Professionalism*	*Competence*
Computer links		Improved follow-up and problem resolution Access to specialists	Improved cognitive control Speed Accuracy
Scheduling and tracking systems	More flexible scheduling to meet personal needs	Improved follow-up and problem resolution	Improved cognitive control Reduced errors Customized information Speed Improved access to information
Teleradiology		Access at inconvenient times or remote locations Access to specialists	Speed Accuracy
Market analysis			Better match with patient needs
Referral systems	Personal attention from friendly staff	Improved follow-up and problem resolution	Improved cognitive control Speed Better match with patient needs
Outbound telemarketing	Personal attention from friendly staff	Improved follow-up and problem resolution	Improved cognitive control Better match with patient needs Better access

Computer technology can increase the patient's "cognitive control" over the care provided, which can increase satisfaction. As Bopp states, "Cognitive control requires that individuals be able to predict the sequence of events and/or understand the implications of these events for themselves."[16] Even though a patient cannot achieve "decisional control," that is, the ability to change the goals and objectives of the encounter,[17] they can achieve some measure of cognitive control, lowering stress.

Table 1.2 Potential Benefits to Referring Physicians of Selected Computer Technologies

Technology	Enhanced Perception of				
	Individualized Care	Convenience to Patient	Meeting Patient Preferences	Communications with Physician	Supporting Practice
Computer links	Customized information	Improved follow-up and problem resolution Speed Access to specialists		Accuracy Improved flow of information	Consult requests Billing information
Scheduling and tracking systems	Customized information	Reduced errors Improved follow-up and problem resolution Speed	More flexible scheduling	Improved flow of information	
Teleradiology	Access to specialists	Speed Reduced patient travel	Access to specialists	Receive images	Remote image interpretation
Market analysis		Improved access	Better match		Market analysis available
Referral systems	Personal attention from staff	Speed Improved follow-up and problem resolution	Better match	Improved flow of information	Increased referrals
Outbound telemarketing	Personal attention from staff	Better access Improved follow-up and problem resolution	Better match	Improved flow of information	Increased referrals

A computer link can increase cognitive control by providing a patient with information, for example, a schedule for outpatient procedures being ordered by their physician at a hospital, a description of the procedures, instructions for any preparations, and the names of those who will be providing treatment. All this can be provided before a patient leaves the referring physician's office.

Since requests for scheduling are recorded and can be individually tracked, computer links offer the potential for improved follow-up and problem resolution. A computer link can be established to specialized physicians and medical facilities, to whom test and other data can be quickly sent, offering improved access to patients.

Computer links can be used to transmit customized information to patients, for example, on the location of a hospital or imaging center, or preparations for a procedure based on the patient's diagnosis. The flow of information to the referring physician can also be improved, for example, by providing access to lab results as soon as they are in a hospital's computer. Computer links can also support a referring physician's practice by allowing requests for specialty consults to move over the link, as well as billing information.

Scheduling systems used with or without a computer link can reduce errors by checking if the necessary resources are available (for example, physicians and equipment) and by checking that the scheduled procedure is not equivalent to one already performed or is not inappropriate for a variety of reasons. Patient perceptions of competence can be improved by providing patients with customized information (via a computer link or through a word processor and the mails) on topics such as how to reach the facility or preparations for a procedure. This can increase the patient's cognitive control of the situation. Scheduling systems can also track each person and procedure to assist in follow-up and problem resolution.

Because the availability of resources can be checked, scheduling systems can provide more flexible scheduling to accommodate patients' personal needs (for example, a family vacation).

Scheduling systems can be combined with a link or word-processing system that generates correspondence to improve the flow of information to the referring physician, for example, concerning when a test has been scheduled or when the results will be ready.

Communication of results

A computer link can improve the speed and accuracy of receiving the results of imaging, lab tests, and other procedures, again by bypassing busy phone systems and by replacing verbal communication of results with the complete text of a report.

Teleradiology systems can transmit x-ray, magnetic resonance imaging (MRI), and computerized tomography (CT) images to a physician over telephone lines for interpretation, reducing some of the travel required to provide this service to a hospital or physician group practice on nights and weekends. Since radiologists can provide an interpretation in their homes or offices, speed and accuracy are improved. The purchase and use of this technology could also improve patient perceptions of the conscientiousness or professionalism of physicians. It can also improve access to the service in areas where radiologists are not available.

Teleradiology can also be used to provide physicians and patients access to the expertise of specialists regardless of where they are located, without always requiring the patient to travel. Patients may no longer need to travel to a regional center for some procedures.

The practices of referring physicians are also supported. Physicians with access to receiving equipment can easily receive images taken elsewhere and can have images produced locally (for example, in a group practice's own imaging center) interpreted by a specialist at a remote site.

Control of the process

Some departmental information systems (for example, for radiology departments) track the utilization of resources. Some use computer-generated bar codes (like the rows of bars on most packaged goods), a device that reads the bar codes, and computer software that records where and when the bar codes were read. Regardless of whether bar codes or another method of recording is used, reports can be prepared on the time needed to perform a task (for example, registering a patient or doing a chest x-ray) and the resources used, offering the possibility of reducing waiting time and, therefore, increasing the speed with which the service is provided. Because the patient's identity, procedure, time, location, and staff involved in rendering a service are recorded, follow-up and problem resolution can be improved.

Such systems also allow for the control of inventory (in the same way a supermarket uses bar codes and a reader at the checkout counter) to assure that items are available when they are needed. The location of films and medical records can also be tracked in this way. A referring physician could benefit from the improved flow of information, such as medical records and images, that results from more accurate tracking of their location.

Reaching Out to Potential Customers

Defining markets

Market analysis systems have been developed that reduce the staff time and skill required by using a computer and software to retrieve, analyze, and produce the tables, maps, and graphs needed to define a market based on where patients and physicians live, their prior use of health services, and demographic and economic characteristics such as age, family size, and income. Financial models are also available to estimate demand and assess the profitability of providing services to these markets.

This can result in improved access to services for these targeted patients and physicians. By carefully identifying the characteristics of the markets it wishes to serve, an organization is able to design services that better match the needs and preferences of these patients and physicians, increasing their satisfaction with services.

Support can be provided to referring physicians by providing them with market analyses that could be useful in targeting groups they wish to serve.

Communicating with and serving potential customers

Once a target market has been identified, and the hospital, physician group, or other provider is prepared to deliver excellent services, communication with the targeted patients and physicians is essential.

Computer-based physician and service referral systems can be used to communicate the availability of services. An offer can be made through various media, including direct mail, to potential patients and physicians to use the referral system. The computer can then be used to match patients and physicians with the physicians and services they feel are appropriate, using many criteria including the type of specialty, office location, hours, and method of payment. The speed with which a patient can be matched is also increased when compared with published sources that are often out-of-date or lack information important to individual patients.

In addition to improving the patient's control of which provider will be used, referral systems can also increase the patient's cognitive control of the subsequent encounter by providing (on the phone or through the mails) information on the qualifications of the physician or other provider, instructions for travel, a description of what will occur during the visit, and information on any preparations that need to be made.

Since the computer stores the name, telephone number, patient problem, and the referral made, improved follow-up and problem resolution are possible. Patients can be called to ask about their progress and their satisfaction with services. Personal attention from friendly staff during the initial call and any follow-up can enhance perceptions that the organization cares.

The flow of information to physicians can be improved when referral systems have word-processing capabilities that provide for automatic correspondence to the physician who has received a referral. Physicians' practices are also supported through increased referrals.

Such referral systems can be combined with computerized outbound telemarketing systems. After contact has been made with the patient in other ways (for example, the patient completes a health questionnaire), an offer of assistance in selecting a physician or service can be made. Such outbound telemarketing systems can also be used alone to market a particular service or services, such as weight control or annual physicals.

The benefits to the patient or physician include improved access to a service or physician because of the information received, and a better match of consumers with providers (i.e., each finds the other desirable on the basis of their objectives and preferences). As a result of personal attention from friendly staff, there may also be an enhanced perception that the sponsoring organization cares about patients and can provide individualized services. An organization that follows up a health awareness campaign with an offer to provide information or a referral to an individual with an identified health risk is likely to be viewed as more professional.

The system also allows for resolving problems that may be faced by patients seeking services. Patients who were registered for a service can also be called back later to determine if the organization can help in resolving any further problems the patient faces (for example, transportation).

As with referral systems, the flow of information to physicians can be improved when telemarketing systems have word-processing capabilities that provide for automatic correspondence to the physician who has received a referral. Physicians' practices are also supported through increased referrals. The cognitive control of the patient is also increased when information is sent on the process of receiving the service, who will provide it, and any preparations that need to be made.

The Employer and Third-Party Payer as Customer

Employers and third-party payers could be viewed as sources of cash, regulators, obstacles to growth and profitability, or customers whose satisfaction is essential. Excellence in the delivery of services to employers and third-party payers is also possible, and computer systems can help.

The potential benefits to the patients listed in Table 1.1 are also important to employers and third-party payers since both benefit from higher levels of employee satisfaction. Some of the benefits listed in Table 1.2 will also be perceived as valuable since employers and third-party payers have some capability through their medical staff or consultants to evaluate medical information. Some potential benefits, however, are distinct from those sought by patients and referring physicians.

Source of information to beneficiaries

A computer link, a referral system, or both can be used to provide information on benefits and the available service network to hospitals and physicians who serve the members of various health maintenance organizations (HMOs), preferred provider organizations (PPOs), and insurance plans, relieving the employer or third-party payer of some of the burden of providing this information.

Source of information on use, cost, and outcomes

A computer link with the employer or third-party payer could also be used to receive and return inquiries, to carry out prior authorization and utilization review, and to share data on utilization and costs, reducing "incurred but not reported" expenses.

Employers and third-party payers can be offered a range of administrative services. Data can be made available to whatever organization is under contract to provide these services, with the results forwarded to the employer or third-party payer. This could increase their sense of control over use and expenditures, while increasing perceptions of the efficiency and professionalism of the hospital or other health care organization.

The Financial Payoff

No attempt will be made to provide an estimate of the dollar payoff of any type of technology. This would require both an estimate of the cost of implementing a technology and the value of benefits received. The features and prices of computer technologies continually change, and health care organizations will need to select from the optional features identified in the chapters in Part II. The financial benefits will depend on the characteristics of the market being served, the actions of competitors, and success in acquiring and using the staff and other resources required for implementation.

Table 1.3 offers suggestions on which technologies an organization might give high priority consideration. It is assumed that the major factors used in deciding whether even to look at a technology are the size of the investment required, the size of the financial payoff, and the level of risk that the payoff will not be achieved. Three categories of organizations are defined in Table 1.3. The groups are not empirically defined, but it is hoped that the reader's organization will fall within one of the three categories.

The rankings given to the technologies are personal judgments of the author, supported by the information contained in Parts II and IV of this book. The rankings were derived by comparing the technologies and do not correspond to any quantitative scale.

The intent here is not to dissuade a health care organization from considering a particular technology, but to help managers efficiently use the resources they have to evaluate various options. Organizations willing to

Table 1.3 Priorities for Evaluation by Category of Health Care Organization

Category 1

Organization desires low investment (a total of $50,000–$100,000 is possible), moderate payoff, low risk.

High-priority technologies:
— physician referral
— scheduling and tracking systems
— fax link to selected physicians
— teleradiology link for evening and weekend coverage by radiologists

Category 2

Organization will make moderate investments ($100,000–500,000 is possible), looking for moderate-to-high payoff, will accept low-to-moderate risk.

Additional high-priority technologies (also see list above):
— market analysis system (assumes additional staff/consultant and data collection costs for a first-time user and additional investment in new services)
— computer link to high-volume physicians
— outbound telemarketing (assumes additional staff and other resources are needed to operate the system and develop new services)

Category 3

Organization will make high investments ($1 million or more not impossible), looking for some high payoffs, will accept moderate-to-high risk.

Additional high-priority technologies:
— computer link with most physicians and other providers that provides support services such as claims processing
— referral system that operates 24 hours per day, seven days a week, offering an assessment of patient problems, service referrals, and information, with the capability to offer services to employers and payers such as specialist referrals and information on insurance coverage
— teleradiology combined with computer storage of most images produced in the organization
— market analysis system linked to a financial system that allows product costing (which is not currently in operation)

devote substantial resources might consider all of them, while a manager with no staff or consultant support might want to focus on those that match a desired level of investment, payoff, and risk.

For example, a manager in a small hospital with no staff available for evaluating technologies might first consider a computer-based physician referral service, where the investment is low, the risk is low, and the payoff is likely to be moderate (assuming that competition among referral services is not high). A large hospital willing to make a larger investment might want to consider a computer link that includes support services for physicians such as claims processing. Here the investment will be high, and the risk will be higher, but the long-range payoff could also be high.

Setting Financial Objectives

The material in this book cannot substitute for a planning process within each organization that includes a consideration of the criteria for investment described later in this chapter and more fully in Part III. It is also important for boards and senior managers (1) to set an appropriate financial objective, and (2) to realize that these computer technologies—because they can and should be part of larger strategies—have payoffs that may be difficult to define precisely.

Written reports and the case studies undertaken suggest that boards of directors and senior management are taking different approaches to examining the profitability or "bottom line" associated with these computer technologies. These approaches are suggested by the financial objectives set, which include:

— higher total return on investment than alternative investments

— breaking even in one to two years

— subsidizing "reasonable" losses

Some organizations view the investment in technology as simply an alternative use of funds. Discounted cash flows are examined for three to five years and compared with other investments, for example stocks, bonds, and money market instruments.

The challenge faced when this approach is used is to separate the impact of the technology from all other changes occurring, especially when a complex strategy for increasing volume and market share is being implemented that involves the offer of new services, improved access, and additional advertising. The impact of only the technology needs to be measured, for example, by matching groups of patients and physicians who did and did not have access to the technology and comparing differences in service utilization.

The added expense and methodological problems associated with pinpointing the impact of the technology lead some organizations to set breaking even on direct costs as an objective. If the capital and operating costs of acquiring and using the technology are offset within one to two years, the investment is considered worthwhile. Because the revenue required is lower, more conservative assumptions can be made about the new service volume that would be needed.

This objective may be particularly attractive when an organization is more concerned with holding market share than growth in volume. The problem involved in determining which current physicians and patients might have gone elsewhere are formidable. Statements by physicians or consumers about what they might do in the future may not be related to actual behavior.

Setting up an experiment to see who does or does not stop using services is difficult since it involves finding two similar groups whose behavior can be watched and denying access to the technology to one group.

A more modest financial objective is that the investment results in subsidies that are "reasonable" in the judgment of the board and senior management. Some organizations are willing to look at limited data on the impact of the technology from other organizations, to measure consumer satisfaction, and to hope that an investment is responsible for both high levels of satisfaction and the retention of physicians and patients. Their focus is on prior estimation of capital and operating costs under various assumptions about use of the technology to increase the confidence of the board and senior management that whatever subsidies are required will not exceed certain levels.

This strategy may be particularly attractive to organizations that wish to provide a service to physicians without stating that a definable financial reward is the objective. It is comparable to low-rent physician office space or free blood pressure screening exams.

Selecting Technologies According to Financial Objectives

If a return on investment is the major criterion for selection, then an organization may want to focus on those technologies that directly produce revenue. For example, outbound telemarketing systems that are used to convert a patient who took a screening exam into a customer for a hospital's outpatient services have an identifiable source of revenue—from the procedures. Where the revenue from a procedure is high, for example, angiography to determine blockage in arteries, the payback from a relatively small number of patients can be high. In contrast, a computer link used for scheduling improves the speed and accuracy of carrying out a routine task. No charge is made for the use of the link. Attributing a financial payoff to the link is more difficult.

A *warning*

While short-run payoffs may be easier to estimate, the long-run payoffs of the computer link may be substantially higher. The loss of the loyalty of a single major admitter to a hospital could be devastating to a hospital's bottom line and far exceed the revenues gained from additional procedures performed as a result of telemarketing.

Which technology should be chosen on the basis of financial payoff? The answer really depends on the relative importance for boards and senior management of short-run vs. long-run payoffs, the level of risk that is considered tolerable, and the financial capability of an organization to make investments with uncertain and only long-run payoffs.

Deciding Which Technologies to Invest In

Criteria for Evaluating Technologies

In addition to the financial analysis just discussed, other criteria that are examined in some detail in Part II can be used by managers to decide if a specific type of technology should be acquired and implemented. They need to be examined in some cases before a financial analysis can be undertaken since they concern assumptions about demand and utilization. The criteria can be grouped into a number of topics.

Who benefits?

Careful assessment of who actually benefits from a technology is needed. If the technology provides benefits to physicians' office staffs while physicians are indifferent, it may not be the technology to invest in to increase referrals or maintain physician loyalty.

Will utilization be affected?

Some benefits may be real and measurable but do not affect the use of services—the ultimate objective. Evidence is needed that benefits of the magnitude provided actually affect behavior.

Is the proposed use ethical and legal?

Some benefits are real and measurable and will affect the use of services, but obtaining them may violate values held by groups in the organization or may violate the law. A hospital could provide physicians with free fax machines, with the expectation that lab and other orders would increase because results would be returned faster. Since the machines cost money, they may be viewed as an additional payment for referrals. This is likely to offend some managers, clinicians, and members of the board of trustees who believe that physicians should not profit from the referral of patients because it alters the role of the physician as an advocate for the patient's welfare. When a Medicare or Medicaid patient is referred, the hospital and physician may also be in violation of the fraud and abuse regulations of the federal government, which bar a financial payment for the referral of a patient. What constitutes fraud and abuse is now being debated in the Congress, the federal bureaucracy, and the courts. Any program that gives physicians free goods or services needs to be reviewed by legal counsel, and by board and staff decision makers.

This is not meant to suggest that providing any goods or services to physicians at less-than-retail prices is automatically unethical or illegal.

Can you sustain the competitive advantage?

Some technologies are more difficult for a competitor to acquire or use, or evolve into complex systems that a competitor will find difficult to duplicate.

Each technology must be evaluated on its ability to produce a sustainable competitive advantage.

Evaluation

Each technology must be justified in the long run by a return to the organization that made the investment. Technologies that come with built-in tools for evaluation, support from the vendor in this activity, or both are therefore desirable.

Implementation

The technologies discussed in this book provide services, and the challenges that arise in implementation are similar to those in the development of any service. A structure and system need to be put in place to provide the service in a way that is consistently excellent. If the organization cannot do this, it needs to forego acquiring the technology. Since technologies require different kinds of resources, this offers one basis for selecting among technologies.

For example, a physician group that cannot provide consistently quick response to requests from referring physicians for consultations may not want to acquire a computer link with those physicians that raises their expectations of fast service. The group may want, however, to acquire a market analysis system that allows it to define its various referral markets by geography, physician type, and patient diagnosis in order to develop an improved marketing strategy. The difference between the two technologies is that one requires continuous, timely response to customers, while the other does not.

Evaluating the Benefits in Your Organization

A technology that delivers extensive benefits in one organization can fail to deliver any in another. The "fit" between technology and organizations is a complex subject that is examined in the in-depth case studies in Part IV of this book.

Putting Technologies Together

The question is not which technology to acquire, but how to select and combine a number of technologies that work together to support a strategy. The technologies described in this book are not multimillion dollar computer systems that are unlikely to be replaced in less than ten years. Rather, many are systems that cost less than $100,000, that perform limited tasks very well, that will need to be enhanced continually, and that are very likely to be obsolete in five years. Health care organizations should therefore begin to think about a "portfolio" of systems and a continuous process of assessing the value of what's new in the computer marketplace.[18]

Critical Factors that Determine Success

Although there are unique characteristics of each hospital, physician group, or other health care organization that must be examined to determine the appropriateness of any specific technology, some things can be learned from examining the experience of other organizations.

This book contains a number of case studies, which suggest some of the factors that may be critical to the successful implementation of the type of computer technologies that are the focus of this book.

The Product Is Service, Not a Technology

The product when each technology is used is service, not files transmitted or messages recorded. Since the use of any computer technology can result in problems or "bugs," especially with systems that are new in the marketplace, there is a tendency to be concerned with those technical problems rather than the more complex question of whether the organization can deliver excellent service. The two issues are related, but not identical.

Although there are many technical issues involved in selecting and implementing computer hardware and software, there is usually some base of expertise and experience for responding to them. It is also clear within a short period of time whether the technical problems have been solved. The challenge for managers is to develop a process for solving the technical problems (with internal and vendor staff working cooperatively and quickly) while getting a larger group of clinical and nontechnical staff ready to deliver excellent service.

Development of a High-Quality Service

The task of consistently delivering excellent service is actually more complex since it requires the cooperation of many people, some of whom have to acquire new skills, knowledge, attitudes, and behavior. The tasks involved in changing the organization, with its unique characteristics and culture, may require several years, while the time required to resolve technical problems is measured in days, weeks, and months.

Providing excellent service will involve the coordination of planning, marketing, and human resources decisions. The need for such coordination is documented in the cases in Part IV. Some of the critical steps in developing a high-quality service have been described earlier and include:

— defining and implementing a service strategy

— developing a structure for services management

— carefully defining expected benefits and continually evaluating the benefits achieved

Service Differentiation

Some thought needs to be given to the capabilities of the competition, what will make a service different enough to attract patients and physicians, and how any competitive advantage will be sustained by continual evolution of the service into something that is very difficult to duplicate.

Some organizations can "leverage" considerable internal resources (for example, data, nationally known physicians) to provide important services and use computer technology to increase the benefits to patients and physicians. Other organizations are trying to use the technology itself to create something valuable, for example, by providing faster and more accurate access to information that could be made available by a number of competing organizations.

But as Porter notes, some organizations can wind up being "stuck in the middle."[19] Although they achieve lower costs, other competitors can produce a service more cheaply. Although they improve service quality (for example, speed in delivering test results), competitors quickly do better. Although they find and serve a new market, a competitor is able to find a way of offering the same market a better or cheaper product.

Differentiation therefore needs to be viewed not as something to be achieved, but as a continuous process that technology can help. As Tom Peters notes, many organizations need to learn to thrive on chaos—continual change in highly competitive markets.[20] Computer technology can be a particularly important survival tool because hardware and software changes continually, offering opportunities for organizations that are capable of exploiting them. In Chapters 2 and 3, a process for continually improving the services provided to patients and physicians through the use of technology is laid out.

Should You Invest?

The decision to invest in a computer technology in order to improve patient and physician satisfaction will depend on many factors, including the quality of the hardware and software, the level of vendor support, and the price in relation to the benefits achieved. The focus of this book is on other issues. In the time it takes to produce a book, information on specific product characteristics, vendor support, and price would become outdated.

What changes more slowly in organizations—including those that deliver health care—is group and individual behavior, strategy, and systems. The focus of this book is therefore on strategy development and implementation, and how computer systems can help.

The answer to the question, "Should you invest?" will depend on a number of factors that are closely examined in this book. Succinctly, the answer is yes if:

— You want to compete on the basis of service quality.

— Your systems are not supporting your staff in producing high levels of physician and patient satisfaction.

— You have the commitment and resources to develop and implement a strategy to achieve service excellence, and to change the systems used in managing services.

How to Use This Book

Organization of the Book

This book has four parts:

— Part I introduces the concept of a service strategy and explains how computer technology can support one.

— Part II discusses the characteristics of a range of individual technologies and their potential benefits.

— Part III provides a set of criteria that could be used to select technologies.

— Part IV presents a number of case studies of health care organizations that have acquired and implemented a few of the technologies.

Audience

The book is intended for presidents or chief executives, strategic planners, marketing directors, and information systems directors in health care organizations, with a focus on hospitals. Not all of the issues each group will be interested in can be addressed in a single book. The focus has therefore been on demonstrating the interrelationships between these various organizational functions, rather than providing all the details needed by these professionals to do their jobs.

It is also hoped that it will give presidents and CEOs a better understanding of the totality of what needs to be accomplished.

Where to Start

The book can be read in a variety of ways, depending on the time and interest of the reader:

— Focus on Part II to understand the diversity of technologies available and their potential benefits.

— Focus on Parts I and IV to understand the process of strategy development and the interrelationships among strategic planning, marketing, and information systems.

— Focus on Parts I and III to prepare a plan to acquire the technologies that includes an evaluation of the organization's needs and the claims being made by vendors.

Regardless of how much of the book is read and in what order, it is hoped that the result is serious consideration of the use of computer technology to achieve service excellence.

Notes

1. Thomas J. Peters and Robert H. Waterman, Jr., *In Search of Excellence: Lessons from America's Best-Run Companies* (New York: Harper and Row, 1982).
2. Karl Albrecht and Ron Zemke, *Service America! Doing Business in the New Economy* (Homewood, Illinois: Dow Jones–Irwin, 1985).
3. Michael E. Porter, *Competitive Advantage: Creating and Sustaining Superior Performance* (New York: Free Press, 1985).
4. Charles J. Austin, *Information Systems for Health Administration, third edition* (Ann Arbor, Michigan: Health Administration Press, 1988).
5. Richard M. Sneider, *Management Guide to Health Care Information Systems* (Rockville, Maryland: Aspen Publishers, 1987).
6. Howard Rowland and Beatrice Rowland, eds., *Hospital Software Sourcebook, second edition* (Rockville, Maryland: Aspen Systems, 1988).
7. John Wilson, Jonathan Joseph, and Otis Port, "Credit Cards: The U.S. Is Taking Its Time Getting 'Smart,'" *Business Week* (February 9, 1987): 88–92.
8. Caroline Ross, Gayle Frommelt, Lisa Hazelwood, and Rowland Chang, "The Role of Expectations in Patient Satisfaction with Medical Care," *Journal of Health Care Marketing* 7, no.4 (December 1987): 16.
9. Avedis Donabedian, *Explorations in Quality Assessment and Monitoring: The Definition of Quality and Approaches to Its Assessment, vol. 1* (Ann Arbor, Michigan: Health Administration Press, 1980).
10. Kenneth Bopp, "How Patients Evaluate the Quality of Ambulatory Medical Encounters: A Marketing Perspective," *Journal of Health Care Marketing* 10, no. 1 (March 1990): 6–15.
11. Robert L. Ludke and Gary S. Levitz, "Referring Physicians: The Forgotten Market," *Health Care Management Review* (Fall 1983): 13–22.
12. James L. Heskett, *Managing in the Service Economy* (Cambridge, Massachusetts: Harvard Business School Press, 1986).
13. Wendy Leebov, *Service Excellence: The Customer Relations Strategy for Health Care* (Chicago: American Hospital Association, 1988).
14. Kristine Peterson, *The Strategic Approach to Quality in Health Care* (Rockville, Maryland: Aspen Publishers, 1988).
15. Addison C. Bennett and Samuel J. Tibbitts, *Maximizing Quality Performance in Healthcare Facilities* (Rockville, Maryland: Aspen Publishers, 1989).
16. Kenneth Bopp, "Value-Added Ambulatory Encounters: A Conceptual Framework," *Journal of Ambulatory Care Management* 12, no. 3 (August 1989): 39.
17. J. R. Averill, "Personal Control over Aversive Stimuli and Its Relationship to Stress," *Psychological Bulletin* 80, no. 4: 286–304.
18. F. Warren McFarlan, "Portfolio Approach to Information Systems," *Harvard Business Review* (September–October 1981): 142–150.
19. Michael E. Porter, *Competitive Advantage*, p. 16.
20. Thomas J. Peters, *Thriving on Chaos* (New York: Knopf, 1987), p. xi.

2.

Service Strategy Development

The process of acquiring computer technology needs to be guided by a larger vision of where the organization is going and the strategies it will use to get there. Otherwise, the organization may be left with a collection of hardware and software that fails to produce the desired results.

In this chapter, a "service strategy" is defined and then illustrated by examining a recent innovation in ambulatory health care—the breast imaging center. This example is also used to illustrate the role of systems in improving service, and how computer technologies in particular might increase patient and referring physician satisfaction. The intent is to demonstrate how computer technology could help implement a service strategy.

Service Strategy—What Does It Mean?

A service strategy is a plan of action to implement what James Heskett calls a "strategic service vision."[1] The basic elements of such a vision are:

— a targeted market
— a well-defined service concept
— a focused operating strategy
— a well-designed service delivery system

The service strategy consists of both this four-part vision and a plan of action to implement it. The plan would consist of specific timetables for staff (for example, for recruitment and training), budgets, contracts, and other elements necessary to develop and operate a service.

138,406

To quickly grasp what Heskett means, let's consider the breast imaging centers that have been developed over the last few years.

Breast Imaging Centers: An Example of a Strategic Service Vision

A number of freestanding and hospital-based breast imaging centers have been established around the country.[2] Exhibit 2.1 is an advertisement for such a center. Although centers vary in how they operate, a pattern can be detected that comes close to the "strategic service vision" discussed by Heskett.

Target Market

The centers share a common target market—women, usually thirty-five and older, whom physicians are counseling to receive a baseline and periodic mammograms, and instruction in breast self-examination.

Service Concept

A service concept describes the way an organization would like to have its service perceived by its customers and employees. Succinctly, the service concept here is fast, professional service by caring, competent professionals in an environment that is comfortable for a middle- and upper middle-class woman.

The service concept is based on a set of assumptions about the benefits being sought by women:

— Technical: accurate diagnosis

— Emotional, psychological: service by professionals who understand the anxiety being felt and who respect the dignity of the individual

— Philosophical, value-related: women deserve not only to be treated as equals to men, but their special needs should be met

Service Package

The benefits are provided by offering what Richard Normann calls a "service package," that is, a set of related items offered to the client.[3] A service package consists of the "core service" and "peripheral services" that enhance the value of the core service. In breast imaging centers, women are offered a service package that consists of a core service—a mammogram (or alternative imaging procedure) of high technical quality—and peripheral services, such as instruction in breast self-examination and health-related information (for example, on risk factors).

Exhibit 2.1 Advertisement for the Mammography Suite at Sibley Memorial Hospital

Mammography At Sibley: Of Women, For Women And By Women.

You probably already know the answer to the question, why have a mammogram?

It's the most reliable method for early detection of breast cancer. It's been estimated that one out of 10 women will get breast cancer. But if the cancer is detected early, there's an approximately 90% cure rate. The American Cancer Society recommends mammography for all women over 35.

One of the best places to have a mammogram is the new Mammography Suite at Sibley Memorial Hospital. Sibley's Woman's Centre is equipped to perform "low-dose" film mammography.

The Suite is a quiet place, separate from our radiology department, a place you'd call elegant. The dressing rooms are comfortable and private, the robes are feminine and lovely.

Everything is done with a woman's needs in mind. Our staff includes women technologists and radiologists. They'll be the only persons with you during your screening.

For a copy of our mammography brochure, or to arrange an appointment, call 537-4795.

For all the right reasons.

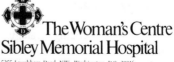 The Woman's Centre
Sibley Memorial Hospital

5255 Loughboro Road, N.W., Washington, D.C. 20016

The attributes of those services are extremely important and include the behavior of staff, the convenient scheduling and speed with which services are provided, and the physical environment in which the services are delivered. Services are provided (1) within a few days of the request, (2) at convenient times, and (3) in a comfortable, professional environment much like a physician's office. Although personnel are efficient, they take the time to provide information and treat the women in a dignified manner. The results are reported to referring physicians within 24 hours. Self-referred women may be provided with the results, offered the opportunity to review the results with a physician affiliated with the center, or both. The objective is to minimize the inconvenience and anxiety associated with the provision of these services, producing psychological benefits. To produce the perceived benefits, both an operating strategy and service delivery system are needed.

Operating Strategy

An operating strategy sets forth the way the service concept will be achieved. It is the product of many decisions about operations, financing, marketing, human resources, and control. The operating strategy here is to focus on:

1. the physical environment in which the patient receives services
2. the selection and training of staff
3. the management of the flow of information to the patient and referring physician

Technical issues like the imaging technology used—although while important—may be given no more attention than in traditional hospital-based imaging departments.

The operating strategy should take advantage of local conditions. This might involve renovating an underutilized section of a hospital (providing, for example, a separate entrance) that would allow sharing of imaging equipment but not patient waiting areas. Female nurses, technologists, and physicians would then be attracted by offering an environment where they had substantial input into the design of the service and how it would be delivered.

Service Delivery System

An ingenious operating strategy intended to provide a service aimed at a particular market segment is useless if the delivery system does not work. Systems that deliver successfully consist of well-thought-out jobs for people with the capabilities and attitudes necessary for successful performance; equipment, facilities, and layouts for effective customer and work flow; and carefully developed procedures aimed at a common set of clearly defined objectives.[4]

In breast imaging centers, the service delivery system that is created to implement this operating strategy calls for, among other things, the use of space separate from areas used by sick patients, the use of female radiology technologists who meet with each woman to explain the procedure and then take the image, and the use of female nurses who take the time to explain and demonstrate breast self-examination. Both interactions occur in private spaces in the center. Waiting rooms are kept small and patients spend little time in them. Supply and demand are carefully monitored and matched to assure that patient scheduling preferences can be met and waiting time at the center minimized. Physicians are called with the results within 24 hours, and written reports and the films arrive within 48 hours by express mail or courier.

Positioning

The service delivery system would help to place the imaging center in the competitive position described in Table 2.1. As Table 2.1 suggests, a comparison of the position of the service in relation to what is offered by competitors is essential. Offering a service that is different from what is being offered by competitors is the only way to assure a competitive advantage. Patients and referring physicians must perceive that they are receiving something of greater value before they will regularly choose one organization's services as opposed to its competitors'.

Need for Market Research

This is a generic strategy since it does not reflect the attitudes, perceptions, and preferences of women in any particular community. The development of a specific strategy should involve local market research. It is important to understand local patient expectations since any long-term competitive advan-

Table 2.1 Market Positioning of a Breast Imaging Center Based on Patient Perceptions

Our Service	*Competitors*
Looks like a prosperous physician's office	Looks like a clinic or ER
Outpatients separate from acutely ill	Acutely ill patients treated in the same area
Caring professionals spend time with patients	Professionals appear busy and unconcerned
Service quickly scheduled	1–2 weeks for an appointment
5–10 minutes waiting time at center	½–1 hour waiting time in department
Results phoned to referring physician in 24 hours	5 + days for results

tage is likely to arise from consistently meeting and exceeding them. An organization that does better than its competitors, but fails to meet consumer expectations, is vulnerable to the entry of a competitor into the market with a service that does.

Market research is needed to confirm both the factors that determine positive perceptions of a service in relationship to what is offered by competitors and the relative influence of the referring physician on the patient's choice of where to receive the service.

The Referring Physician

Since a physician must make the referral for services, it is important to consider what factors might affect the physician's choice. Table 2.2 uses the concepts described in Table 1.2 to suggest how a breast imaging center might attempt to position itself in order to receive a higher number of referrals from physicians.

The Importance of Systems

Systems are one of the "Seven S's" (i.e., structure, systems, style, staff, skills, strategy, and shared values) described by Tom Peters and Robert Waterman, Jr.,[5] as essential for achieving service excellence. The failure of systems to support health professionals—and the resulting failure to meet patient and physician expectations—is a common topic of discussion in many

Table 2.2   Market Positioning of a Breast Imaging Center Based on Referring Physician Perceptions

Our Service	*Competitors*
Individualized care Customized communication sent automatically	Patients must call to get generic material
Convenience to Patient Service quickly scheduled; 5–10 minutes waiting time at center	1–2 weeks for an appointment; ½–1 hour waiting time in department
Meeting Patient Preferences Day and hour preferences usually met	Book only for current calendar month with few choices of day and hour
Communications with Physician Results to referring physician in 24 hours	5 + days for results
Supporting Practice Efficient service enhances physician image	Inconvenient service hurts physician image

health care organizations. Typical of the situations related to systems that occur are the following:

— The patient arrives, but the medical record is not available at the clinic/office.

— Patient waiting time in the office lengthens, but there is no system for analyzing or dealing with whatever is causing the problem.

— A physician or office staff member cannot get through on the telephone to schedule a service.

Each situation represents a "moment of truth" for the health care organization, a term borrowed from bullfighting by Jan Carlzon, the president of SAS Airlines, to describe those contacts with the customer that shape attitudes toward the company and the desire to use its services.[6]

It is testimony to the low expectations of both patients and physicians that they regularly face these situations and continue to use an organization's services. The opportunity for those health care organizations desiring to both survive and grow is to meet and raise those expectations in order to achieve a formidable competitive advantage in the market place.

There are reasons other than market share and profits to do so. Many, if not most, health care professionals are instructed that their primary mission is to serve. Failing to serve a patient or physician is frustrating. Frustrated people are less productive and are more likely to leave their jobs, and even careers. As hospitals and other health care organizations know, replacing nurses with full-time or temporary staff is expensive and time-consuming. As Karl Albrecht notes

> As we have known for centuries, mobilizing people to constructive action is less a matter of motivating them than it is of getting rid of the factors that *demotivate* them. So, if we're going to make service excellence the strategic focus of a business, we have to go to work on the organization itself. We have to find and eliminate the demotivators, the disincentives.[7]

There are many reasons for staff turnover and recruitment problems; the failure to provide good service because of systems that do not support staff is one of them. This includes the failure to fix the problems mentioned earlier— to implement a system for tracking the location of medical records, to monitor patient waiting time and find the causes of delays, and to relieve overburdened telephone systems by using other modes of communication.

Information Technologies for Service Enhancement

Technologies exist that have the potential to improve patient and physician satisfaction with services and to help achieve a desired market position.

Examples relevant to the service strategy of breast imaging centers include the following:

— Hardware and software for linking the physician to a health care organization that allow the transmittal of patient information, the scheduling of services, and the use of data available in the health care organization.

— Systems that allow for tracking the patient through the process of scheduling and receiving care to detect deviations from standards that require correction by managers. Some systems use the data stored and word-processing software to produce customized correspondence to the patient and referring physician.

A link with the physician's office facilitates communications with the physician, and ultimately the patient. More detailed information on such links appears in Part II, and case studies on the implementation of computer links appear in Part III.

Tables 1.1 and 1.2 summarize the potential benefits to patients and referring physicians of such computer links. Organizations that implement such links often do so with the hope that a physician and patient will become dependent on the flow of information provided and will therefore continue to use the services of the organization.[8] Because of the competitive advantages they can provide, computer links are one example of a "strategic" application of information technology.[9]

Systems for monitoring the process of providing services do not offer the physician and patient additional information, but instead provide managers and front-line employees with information on performance. The physician and patient gain through receiving a service that provides greater benefits, for example, takes less time to receive.

Using Computer Technologies to Implement a Service Strategy

These technologies could be used to help implement a service strategy by assisting front-line staff such as nurses and physicians to meet and exceed patient and physician expectations.

Table 2.3 shows a number of technologies that could be added to the service delivery system to enhance the quality of the service provided in a breast imaging center and to achieve the market position described in Tables 2.1 and 2.2. Each service enhancement could allow the radiology department or freestanding imaging center to differentiate itself from a competitor. Which enhancement should be selected will depend on the department's or

Table 2.3 Uses of Technology to Improve Service Quality in a Breast Imaging Center

		Potential Impact*	
Service Enhancement	*Technology Added*	*Improved Patient Perception of Staff*	*Improved Physician Perception of*
Quick scheduling of procedure	Service scheduling and confirmation via computer link with physician's office	Competence	Convenience to patient
Unhurried, but efficient, provision of service	Patient scheduling system that monitors and projects patient flow and allows for corrections (for example, call patient to delay departure or reschedule the same day)	Caring	Convenience to patient
Quick reporting of results	Results available (or automatically transmitted) via computer	Competence Caring	Communications with physician
Greater patient knowledge	Customized letter produced by computer with details on where, when, and how the services will be provided	Competence	Individualized care

*See Table 1.1

center's desired market position, as described in a table such as Tables 2.1 and 2.2. A technology would then be selected on the basis of its ability to significantly contribute to achieving the desired change, for example, quicker reporting of results.

Certain technologies will therefore be extremely important for some departments or centers, but not for others. If market research (for example, surveys or informal interviews with patients and referring physicians) suggests that expectations concerning the speed with which results are received are being met—and that competitors do not offer better service—the transmission of results via computer might not be a worthwhile investment.

In other environments, transmission of reports via computer could offer a significant competitive advantage by differentiating the department/center from its competitors. Whether it is worthwhile to make the investment will depend on the value that patients and referring physicians attach to receiving information earlier, an important subject for market research. The criteria for acquiring a technology are discussed in greater detail in Part III.

The major point here is that computer technology can make a contribution to implementing a service strategy and help an organization to attain a competitive advantage in a specific market.

Does Technology Dehumanize the Delivery of Health Services?

Instead of dehumanizing the process of delivering services, computer technology offers the potential for customizing, enhancing, and speeding up communications. The technology can assist physicians, nurses, and other staff in acting in a way that is perceived as more caring, competent, and professional.

Patients who receive health services have gotten used to very limited communications, delays in scheduling, and other problems. Technology offers the potential of improving the "high touch" as well as the "high tech" elements of health care, as described by John Naisbitt in *Megatrends*:

> Whenever a new technology is introduced into society, there must be a counterbalancing human response that is high touch, or the technology is rejected. The more high tech, the more high touch. And that translates into more personal service.[10]

On the other hand, the arrival of communications by computer, among other innovations, could depersonalize the delivery of services. The choice will be made by the health care organizations who choose and operate the technology.

Notes

An earlier version of parts of this chapter appeared as Roger Kropf, "Computerizing for a Competitive Edge," *Administrative Radiology* (November 1988): 108, 110, 112.

1. James L. Heskett, *Managing in the Service Economy* (Cambridge, Massachusetts: Harvard Business School Press, 1986), p. 7.
2. C. O. Brown, "Breast Evaluation Center, Phoenix," *Medicenter Management* (April 1986); K. Seago, "Breast Imaging Centers and Patient Emotions: Niceness Counts," *Applied Radiology* (November–December 1986); and E. Walker, "Mammography: Linking the Referring Physician," *Administrative Radiology* (March 1987).
3. Richard Normann, *Service Management: Strategy and Leadership in Service Businesses* (Chichester, England: John Wiley & Sons, 1984).
4. Heskett, *Service Economy*, p. 20.
5. Thomas J. Peters and Robert H. Waterman, Jr., *In Search of Excellence: Lessons from America's Best-Run Companies* (New York: Harper and Row, 1982).
6. Jan Carlzon, *Moments of Truth* (Cambridge, Massachusetts: Ballinger, 1987).
7. Karl Albrecht, *At America's Service* (Homewood, Illinois: Dow Jones–Irwin, 1988).
8. Alexander J. Szafran and Roger Kropf, "Strategic Uses of Teleradiology," *Radiology Management* 10, no. 2 (Spring 1988).
9. See, for example: Michael E. Porter and V. Millar, "How Information Gives You a Competitive Advantage," *Harvard Business Review* (July–August 1985) and E. W. McFarlan, "Information Technology Changes the Way You Compete," *Harvard Business Review* (May–June 1984).
10. John Naisbitt, *Megatrends: Ten New Directions Transforming Our Lives* (New York: Warner Books, 1982).

3.

Creative Thinking about the Use of Computer Technology

Finding Ways to Support a Specific Service Strategy

There are a number of ways to generate ideas about the use of computer technology to pursue a strategy of service excellence. Searching for examples in magazines, journals, and vendor product descriptions is one method. The examples that are provided, however, may not reflect the needs of a specific service strategy, that is, a specific target market, service concept, operating strategy, and service delivery system.

To support a specific service strategy, some more systematic method for generating ideas is needed. There are a number of possibilities. Shostack has suggested the use of "service blueprints," that is, detailed flowcharts that depict the steps involved in providing a service and assist in identifying where problems may arise.[1] Corrective action—including the use of computer systems—can then be taken.

Marketing professionals have used the techniques and concepts of psychology to study what factors contribute to the decision to purchase a service.[2] Some of those factors, for example, the quantity and quality of the information received from a physician, could be affected by the use of computer technology.

In this chapter, another method is presented that is more closely related to economics than psychology. It is the use of a "value chain" to generate ideas on how to increase the value of a service to the patient and physician, and the selection of a strategy to differentiate a service from what is being provided by competitors. After defining a value chain and three generic strategies, two examples of how to apply the method to improving health services are presented.

Value Chains

Michael Porter has used concepts from economics to explain how a firm might achieve a competitive advantage by providing greater value to the customer. He has identified the collection of activities that create value for a firm's customers and called it a "value chain."[3]

A chain is composed of economically and technologically distinct activities and can be divided into primary and support activities. Primary activities are "the activities involved in the physical creation of the product and its sale and transfer to the buyer as well as after-sale assistance."[4] This includes inbound logistics (activities associated with receiving, storing, and disseminating inputs to the product), operations, outbound logistics (activities associated with collecting, storing, and physically distributing the product to buyers), marketing and sales, and service. "Support activities support the primary activities and each other by providing purchased inputs, technology, human resources and various firmwide functions."[5] This includes firm infrastructure, human resources management, technology development, and procurement.

The firm's value chain is embedded in a larger stream of activities called the value system, which includes the value chains of suppliers, distribution channels, and buyers. The chains are interrelated; for example, value activities of the producing firm can affect the value created for both distribution channels and buyers. By increasing the value received anywhere along the customer's chain, a firm increases the chances that the customer will be willing to pay a premium price, or will use a product in greater volumes, that is, that it will obtain a competitive advantage.

Porter has applied his concepts to the production of goods, not health services. To understand how they might apply to health services, the value chains of patients and referring physicians who use several types of health services will be described. Before doing that, Porter's definition of the generic strategies available for competing in a market will be presented. The selection of a strategy is a critical step for a firm since it will determine its overall objective in increasing value along the customer's value chain.

Generic Competitive Strategies

Michael Porter suggests that there are fundamentally two types of competitive strategies—differentiation and cost leadership.[6] In a differentiation strategy, an organization seeks to be unique along some dimensions that are valued by many segments of the market. In a cost leadership strategy, a firm sets out to become the low-cost producer in its industry. Consider the following examples:

— The Arizona Heart Institute in Phoenix has a "HARTLINE" (1-800-345-HART), which patients can use to schedule airline connections into Phoenix, hotel accommodations, and transportation to and from the airport.

— Gettysburg Hospital was able to reduce the charge for a mammogram by developing a uniform medical history questionnaire and breast examination diagram that could be completed by the referring physician, eliminating the need to complete these steps at the time the image was taken and lowering the cost to the hospital.[7]

In Porter's terms, the Arizona Heart Institute is using a differentiation strategy, and Gettysburg Hospital has taken actions that could lead to cost leadership. HARTLINE makes the services of the Arizona Heart Institute different, and more valuable, for out-of-town patients who need a wide range of cardiac-related procedures. Gettysburg Hospital has achieved a reduction in cost that could lead to its being the low-cost mammography center in its community.

Differentiation

Certain characteristics of a service are valued by many segments of the market, for example, quick and easy scheduling of an appointment. By applying information systems technology, a health care organization could differentiate itself from a competitor, resulting in higher volumes of service or the ability to charge a higher price.

Cost Leadership

Cost leadership is the ability to produce a service at the lowest cost. Porter believes that ten major "cost drivers" determine the cost behavior of value activities: economies of scale, learning, the pattern of capacity utilization, linkages, interrelationships, integration, timing, discretionary policies, location, and institutional factors.[8]

A cost advantage can be gained in two major ways—by controlling the cost drivers or by reconfiguring the value chain.[9] Health care organizations can take numerous actions to control cost drivers. For example, contracts with an HMO or PPO could allow a clinical laboratory to achieve economies of scale that would not be possible at lower levels of utilization.

Gettysburg Hospital was able to decrease the charge for a mammography by $40 by reconfiguring its value chain. It eliminated the need for its staff to complete a medical history questionnaire and breast examination diagram, lowering its costs.[10]

For the patient and referring physician, price is more important than a health care organization's costs. By focusing on the customer's value chain, creative ways of increasing customer value by lowering price (in both time and money) could be developed. For example, a package rate for accommodations and meals for out-of-town patients could be developed by securing discounts from hotels and restaurants. This would cost a health care organization nothing, especially if a local travel agency provides the staff, but secure a real price reduction for receiving services for the patient.

Focus

Differentiation and cost leadership strategies can be used in a few or a large number of the market segments that a health care organization is trying to reach. When an organization seeks a cost advantage in a target segment, it is pursuing a *cost focus* strategy. In *differentiation focus*, a firm seeks differentiation in a target segment.[11]

By offering travel services, the Arizona Heart Institute is enhancing the service package of only a segment of its market (i.e., out-of-town residents). If all of its service enhancements are offered to only selected segments of its market, it is pursuing a differentiation focus strategy, that is, it is attempting to offer a different and valued service to just some of the patients it is trying to serve. If it offers a service package intended to be attractive to all patients, it is pursuing a differentiation strategy.

Likewise, if Gettysburg Hospital attempts to achieve the lowest cost of any organization just for mammographies, it is pursuing a cost focus strategy. If it extends its efforts to all services, it can be said to pursue cost leadership.

Richard Normann notes that there are several possible approaches to individualizing the service package. The first is the development of a set of preconceived and standardized service packages, each reflecting the needs of one well-understood customer segment. The second is the assignment of individual contact people who can vary the service package provided. The third is "computerized individualization," in which the service package offered depends on the market segment to which a customer is assigned, and the computer is used to put together mailings, schedules, and other information that presumably reflects the customer's needs.[12]

A special mailing to patients traveling a distance (identified by looking at their zip code) is an example of a service that could be computerized. Some of the special needs of children and parents when a child receives services such as cancer treatment might be met either through a standardized package or with an individual contact person.

Deciding on What Strategy to Pursue

Defining current strategy

These categories can be used to generate ideas about alternative strategies that a health care organization could pursue. An important step is to define the current strategy of the organization and its major competitors.[13] The strategies may or may not have been formally adopted—or ever put down on paper.

Describing how markets are segmented is critically important. What distinctions between patients are considered important? Age? Insurance coverage? Diagnosis? Procedure? What groups of referring physicians are treated as separate in terms of their importance to the organization? Can they be defined by specialty? By age? By office location?

The next step is to determine the current basis of competition. Is there price competition? Is there competition to offer the latest technology? Are amenities used to attract patients and physicians?

The result of this stage should be an understanding of the strategies being pursued using the concepts of differentiation, cost leadership, cost focus, and differentiation focus described earlier. Some examples are the following:

— Differentiation: We offer referring physicians the fastest turnaround on reports of anyone in the community.

— Cost leadership: We achieve economies of scale by increasing volume for a select number of procedures and not offering others where volume is likely to be low. We use the low costs to generate higher profits for some services, and increase/hold market share by offering substantial discounts for volume purchasers when price competition develops.

— Cost focus: We provide the lowest-cost lens implantation services in the community by offering volume-related discounts that allow fixed costs to be spread over a larger number of procedures.

— Differentiation focus: We offer customized services for families of children with cancer that include education about the health effects of imaging procedures.

Setting future strategy

To set future strategy, some predictions about the environment must be made. Of particular importance is deciding on the extent to which price will play a role in the decisions of patients and referring physicians.

Differentiation or cost leadership?   Market conditions vary widely. In areas where PPOs and HMOs have been (or are expected to be) successful in achieving high market share, competition over price may make it necessary to pursue a cost leadership strategy. If costs can be lowered, a health care organization has the ability to either increase profits or survive the next wave of price reductions forced by competition. As the example of Gettysburg Hospital suggests, cost reductions can be achieved not only through productivity improvements and price reductions by suppliers, but also through a rethinking of what the components of the service package are.

If price is likely to stay less important, as in areas where there are high income levels and less market penetration of managed care plans, then differentiating the organization from competitors may be the most important action to take to develop a competitive advantage. What do patients and physicians want that we and our competitors aren't giving them? Are there needs that are widely shared by many of the patients and referring physicians we serve?

Market research may suggest how a service could be enhanced to differentiate it from competitors. Some examples include the following:

— When referring physicians tell us that turnaround time on reports is a problem, computer "mailboxes" can be established to give physicians access to results as soon as specialists (for example, a pathologist or radiologist) have approved a report.

— When patients tell us that they don't receive enough information about imaging procedures, customized letters that include material on the procedure to be done can be prepared by a computer and sent to all outpatients.

Focus on a few market segments?   It is not always possible or desirable to compete for all segments of the market, either on the basis of price or service quality. In this case, a focus on one or more segments may be the best strategy. Which segments? This will depend on the nature of services being offered by competitors, the capabilities of the organization, the needs of patients and physicians, and the size of the market segments under consideration.

It is critically important to first segment the market by relevant variables such as diagnosis, procedure, age, and insurance coverage. Whom have we and our competitors focused on in the past, by intention or without much forethought? Who has not been served? The number of possibilities is large. Cancer treatment may have been important for the department, but the focus has been on adults, and not children. Who *does* focus on children? Is the market large enough to warrant special services? The current emphasis on women's services is the product of this kind of questioning that has proved highly profitable for some organizations and has greatly improved the quality of service for some women.

If a market segment can be found that others are not serving, and that is potentially large in relationship to the resources required to serve it, then a cost focus or differentiation focus strategy could be pursued. Are consumers or third-party payers price sensitive? Even if they are not, the health care organization may want to pursue a cost focus strategy in order to serve the market at the same prices, but with a higher level of profitability. Some of the profits can be passed on later to consumers in the form of lower prices or used to improve the quality of services.

A differentiation focus strategy can be pursued when consumers are not highly price sensitive, that is, when they will pay more for a service that they perceive to be of a higher value. But mistakes can be made in predicting how patients and physicians decide on which services to use. Imaging departments/centers that bought dual-photon densitometers assumed that patients would be willing to pay the higher price for what physicians believed was more accurate results.[14] There are several explanations for reports that such equipment is not utilized to capacity:

1. Women are more price sensitive than expected.
2. Women did not value the higher accuracy, especially since it required a significantly greater exposure to radiation.
3. Both of the above.

An understanding of the needs and desires of the customer—both the patient and referring physician—is critically important in avoiding situations where new services fail to achieve projected utilization.[15]

Although obtaining state-of-the-art technology and enhancing the quality of clinical services will remain important competitive strategies, managers of health care organizations should also consider the other strategies that are available. Thinking about the generic competitive strategies of differentiation and cost leadership will help in both the initial brainstorming for ideas and setting priorities for the market research that follows.

Value Chains of Patients and Referring Physicians

The generic strategy selected determines the basic approach to be used in enhancing both the core and peripheral services offered to patients and referring physicians. After the value chains are described, each activity on the chain can be examined to determine what changes could be made to contribute to differentiating the service package from what is being offered by a competitor, or to achieve a cost leadership position. A decision on market scope, that is, the number of segments of the market to be served, also needs to be made to determine if a cost or differentiation focus strategy is to be pursued.

The use of computer technology to increase buyer value will be emphasized in the following examples. As Porter notes, "Information systems technology is particularly pervasive in the value chain, since every value activity creates and uses information."[16]

To gain a competitive advantage, a manager needs to understand the customer's value chain and develop a service package that will be rated as superior to competitors. Customers can assign different values to parts of the package, making some of them "core services" and others "peripheral services." When there is little difference between the core services of competing companies, customer choices may be determined by the availability of peripheral services. Service packages are evaluated on the basis of prior experience and promises.[17]

The potential for improving services offered (1) by specialists in their offices (for example, cardiologists) and (2) to outpatients by hospital radiology departments and freestanding imaging centers will be examined. The methodology could, of course, be extended to a variety of other services.

Service Enhancement in Office-Based Specialty Health Care

The first step in using value chains to generate ideas on how to enhance services is to write down what are the economically and technologically distinct activities that a patient or referring physician must engage in to receive services. The emphasis here is not on the decisions to be made, but the activities that generate a cost (either in money or in opportunity costs, that is, the cost of not engaging in an alternative activity like going to work) or require a new set of resources.

Value Chain of the Patient

The activities that patients engage in to receive many office-based specialty services might be described as follows:

> Visit to primary care physician→Schedule visit to specialist→ Travel to specialist → Office visit → Return home → Travel to site of further tests → Receive tests/procedures → Return home → Travel for return visit to specialist → Visit → Return home → Travel to primary care physician → Visit → Return home → Payment for services → Request reimbursement → Reimbursement received

Other activities could be required depending on the nature of the illness and the number of diagnostic and therapeutic services required.

Increasing Value to the Patient

The value of services to the patient could be increased at many points along this chain. Ideas can be generated by staff discussion of their perception of the difficulties patients face at a particular point, through focus groups or surveys of patients, or by observation. The creative task is then to think of ways that computer technology might enhance value along the chain.

One approach is to look at the categories described in Table 1.1 and ask if the technology could produce a specific benefit (for example, an enhanced perception of competence) as a result of an outcome of the use of the technology (for example, the speed with which information is transferred). Ideas can be solicited from staff individually or in group brainstorming sessions.

The same methods for idea generation used in a general quality improvement program can be applied here. The difference is that staff need to be knowledgeable about the characteristics and potential benefits of computer technology not currently in use. Consultants, peers in other organizations, and hopefully this book can help.

Some examples of the outcome of such an idea generation process include the following.

Differentiation strategies

Office visit. Show concern about patient waiting time by telling patients how long the wait is likely to be when they arrive, and by monitoring patient waiting time and reducing it. A computer-based scheduling system can capture the necessary data and produce real-time (i.e., accurate at any time) management reports.

Request payment. Offer assistance in completing insurance forms. Use a computer link with hospitals, labs, and imaging centers to provide patients with the information they need to request reimbursement faster.

Receive tests/procedures. Develop a formal education program to educate patients so that they obtain greater "cognitive control" (i.e., a perception that the person is in control resulting from greater knowledge). Use a computer-based scheduling system that incorporates a word processor to produce customized letters and packets of materials that are relevant to a patient's problem or the tests/procedures they are to receive.

Cost leadership

Schedule visit. Ask patient and physician to complete a standardized visit questionnaire when a visit is scheduled to assure that the appropriate resources are available when the patient visits. If the patient is concerned about the condition of their heart or the physician feels that such an evaluation is desirable, the equipment for a cardiac stress test may be needed. Knowing this beforehand can avoid situations where the equipment is needed by another patient at the same time—requiring that one patient return at a later time. Costs are lowered because resources (for example, staff and equipment) are scheduled to produce higher productivity without inconvenience to the patient. A computer link allows the questionnaire to be completed in the primary care physician's office and transmitted instantly, resulting in faster scheduling.

Payment for services.   Coverage verification and claims submission using a computer link reduces bad debts, lowering costs, while allowing patients to determine their out-of-pocket expenses, if any.

Focus strategies

Receive tests/procedures.   Analyze data on patient problem and diagnosis and identify high-use categories. Identify special needs of these patients. For example, free pick-up and return in an appropriately equipped van could be offered to disabled outpatients. (This is an example of a differentiation focus strategy.)

Payment for services.   Establish a computer link for eligibility determination and claims submission to the HMO/PPO who provides the greatest number of patients to the practice. (This is an example of a cost focus strategy.)

Value Chain of the Referring Physician

The value chain of the referring physician might be described as follows:

> Examine patient → Write referral order → Receive results from
> specialist → Patient visit → Request payment from patient → Complete
> insurance forms → Payment received

Increasing Value for the Referring Physician

Differentiation strategies

Write referral order.   Provide patients with information on preparations to take before a procedure is performed. Use a computer-based scheduling system to identify what information patients need and to customize mailings.

Receive results.   Use a computer link or a word-processing system tied to a computer to provide fast reporting of the results of a consultation.

Cost leadership

The cost (and price charged) for services in the specialty practice does not enhance the value of services to the referring physician directly. To the extent that the patient's out-of-pocket costs for specialty care are lowered, the referring physician will benefit indirectly by having patients who are more satisfied with how their care is being managed. This could lead to greater patient loyalty and additional patients.

If the costs to the specialty practice can be reduced while the charges collected remain the same, profits will increase. This benefits the specialty practice, but not the patient or referring physician.

Write referral order.   A computer link can be used to transmit billing and other information to the specialist's office that allows for verification of insurance coverage prior to the patient's visit. If services are not fully covered, payment arrangements can be made that reduce bad debts and reduce patient dissatisfaction as a result of unexpected bills.

Focus strategies

1. Write referral order.   Using a data base from the practice's scheduling system, analyze the types of patients referred by individual physicians. When a pattern is identified (for example, a high number of elderly, arthritic patients), send relevant professionals materials with the compliments of the specialist. This might include articles on the role of exercise and physical therapy in managing arthritis, or on new drugs for managing pain. Use the word-processing system to generate customized letters. (This is an example of a differentiation focus strategy.)

2. Write referral order.   Using a data base from the scheduling system, analyze the patterns of referral by time and day of the week for which an appointment was requested. Contact certain physicians and offer reduced prices or faster scheduling of patients for an appointment if they encourage patients to request appointments at times of lower demand. By smoothing out demand, the resources of the specialty practice may be more effectively used, reducing costs or avoiding the cost of additional staff and equipment. (This is an example of a cost focus strategy.)

Service Enhancement in Outpatient Radiology Services

The second example concerns outpatient radiology services, one of the services to which a specialist or primary care physician might refer a patient. Rather than organizing potential service enhancements by type of strategy, they are organized by value activity. Either approach to generating ideas is equally valid, and the choice depends on what is easier or more productive for managers and staff.

Value Chain of the Patient

The activities that patients engage in to receive an outpatient radiology procedure might be described as follows:

Referral → Schedule procedure → Travel to site → Film/image taken → Return home → Receive results from referring physician → Receive bill → Payment → Request reimbursement → Reimbursement received

Each activity along the value chain can be examined to determine what actions increase the value received by patients. A few examples are provided below.

Increasing Value for the Patient

Schedule procedure

By establishing a computer link between the offices of high-volume referring physicians and the radiology service, the time needed to schedule an appointment could be reduced. A computer link could also allow the immediate delivery of a printed set of instructions to patients on how to prepare for the test, how to reach the radiology service facility, and what to expect when they arrive. The computer could print out personalized instructions specific to the procedure to be performed. A patient who is going to have an MRI, for example, could be told to wear a jogging suit without metal zippers, avoiding the need to disrobe upon arrival. Information on MRI and the specific images to be taken could also be provided, along with a letter welcoming the patient to the imaging facility.

Travel to site

Patients who must travel long distances for services may need overnight hotel accommodations. Data on patient address can be used to segment patients by estimated travel time. Information on local hotels can then be mailed directly to patients who are coming from a distant community. A word-processing system can produce customized letters.

A package rate that includes meals and hotel accommodations for the patient and a companion might also be offered to lower the cost of the service to the patient. If local hotels and restaurants will provide a discount, the price to the patient can be lowered without lowering the revenue received by the radiology service.

Film/image taken

An analysis of past utilization may detect a growing number of patients with a particular problem/complaint or diagnosis. The special needs of those patients might be explored. A growing number of pediatric oncology patients, for example, may suggest the need for a special orientation for parents and children about radiology services to ease concern about their effects on young children. This analysis will increase the value of the "film/image taken" segment of the value chain, and may even increase the value of the "receive results" segment by increasing confidence in the ability of the radiologist and other personnel.

Receive results

An analysis of the time it takes for the referring physician to receive the radiologist's report for a procedure may suggest that improved turnaround time would increase the value of the service and differentiate the service from competitors. Putting the written report in a computer data base that can be accessed by the office computer of a referring physician immediately after transcription might dramatically improve turnaround time.

Choice of generic strategy

Table 3.1 categorizes each service change by type of strategy. Managers can use a similar matrix to generate ideas for further changes in the service package. Each value activity could be discussed, as well as the appropriateness of each generic type of strategy. Particular service changes to implement that strategy can then be suggested.

Value Chain of the Referring Physician

The process of generating ideas for improving the value received by referring physicians is not different in its concepts or methodology. We will provide only a few examples of what service changes might be considered, which is not intended to suggest that studying the value chain of the referring physi-

Table 3.1 Service Changes Categorized by Type of Strategy

Patient Value Activity	Service Change	Strategy Type
Schedule procedure	On-line computer scheduling and information dissemination	Differentiation
Travel to site	Hotel and travel information sent to home	Differentiation focus
	Package rate	Cost focus
Film/image taken	Special orientation for particular patient groups	Differentiation focus
Receive results	Written report available in central data base immediately after transcription	Differentiation

cian is less important. The referring physician is likely to have a considerable influence on what services are requested and where they are received.

The value chain of a referring physician might be described as follows:

Examination → Referral → Receive results → Diagnosis → Treatment or referral → Billing → Payment received

The organization that provides a radiology service might increase the value of its services at one or more points in the value chain.

Increasing Value for the Referring Physician

Referral

Analysis of existing data bases on the procedures requested by specific physicians and the subsequent diagnoses may suggest that physicians are not considering alternative procedures with greater diagnostic value. These physicians could be offered the opportunity to consult with a specialist over the telephone on which procedures to request, increasing the value of services at both the "referral" and "diagnosis" segments of the value chain. The service package can therefore be customized by an individual contact person.

For example, when an analysis shows that dentists are ordering CT scans for patients who are complaining of headaches, the dentists could be offered the opportunity to consult with a specialist on the appropriateness of ordering MRI scans to detect the causes of the problem, including disorders of the temporomandibular joint (TMJ).

Treatment

An analysis of diagnoses made may reveal that individual physicians are treating significant numbers of patients who could be expected to use certain types of therapeutic services. Personal contact could then be made with these physicians to offer assistance in scheduling such services, including inpatient admissions, surgery, and specialized nuclear medicine or drug treatments, increasing value at the "treatment" segment of the value chain. A standardized package of services could be developed, or the package could be customized by an individual contact person. A computer might customize the mailing of educational material to physicians to reflect what is known about the individual physician's qualifications and case mix.

Other Tasks Before Changes Are Made

Market Research

Before time and money are spent to change a service package, the decision process of patients and referring physicians should be explored. Do patients give equal weight to each activity in their value chain, for example, or are some activities more important than others in determining utilization? Market research is needed, which can include both the analysis of any existing data, as well as new data collection using a variety of techniques such as focus groups and telephone or personal surveys.

Other Value Chains

The value chain of the specialty practice or imaging center itself has not been described since the purpose was not to improve their production process, but to increase value as perceived by referring physicians and patients. Once managers understand how value is created for the patient and referring physician, they then need to go back and understand how the value chain of their organization does or does not increase that value.

The value chains of other organizations (including employers, insurance companies, PPOs, and HMOs) who buy services, or the value chains of physicians who work with or for a health care organization, were also not described. Consideration of physician value chains (for example, radiologists) would be especially important in communities where hospitals and imaging centers must compete for the services of these physicians.

Service Excellence as a Competitive Strategy

Service excellence—meeting and exceeding customer expectations concerning services—is not another generic competitive strategy, but a variation on several of those just discussed. A health care organization that seeks to attain service excellence faces the same generic questions:

Differentiation or cost leadership?   Do patients and physicians value cost or unique features of the service that distinguish it from what is provided by competitors? Would lower prices or enhancements in the service influence them to choose one organization over another?

Focus on a few market segments?   Should the organization try for excellence in the services provided to all segments of the market, or just a few? Should we seek to differentiate what we provide to a few segments, or seek to lower prices?

Choices must be made, unless the organization believes it can manage *all* the elements involved in delivering *all* services to *all* the patients and physicians it serves—an unrealistic goal for most organizations.

As Porter notes, some organizations can wind up being "stuck in the middle."[18] Although they achieve lower costs, other competitors can produce a service more cheaply. Although they improve service quality (for example, speed in delivering test results), competitors quickly do better. Although they find and serve a new market, a competitor is able to find a way of offering the same market a better or cheaper product.

Realistically, a health care organization needs to consider the development of a "service strategy" with much more limited and attainable objectives. In an organization that provides a wide range of services to many market segments, this probably means establishing a strategy at the product, unit, or departmental level. As the strategy succeeds, the organization can develop strategies for other products/units/departments.

Michael Porter and Victor Millar,[19] as well as Charles Wiseman,[20] have recognized the importance of information systems in developing a competitive advantage and recommend a formal process within firms of evaluating the information systems used to support each activity.

Careful, continuous evaluation of what value is being created for patients and physicians is essential. Karl Albrecht and Ron Zemke believe that when no one is in charge of the cycle of service (or service package as Normann describes it), the result is a regression to mediocrity. They believe each contact with the consumer is a "moment of truth" that must be managed.[21] In an increasingly competitive environment, fewer health care institutions can afford the regression to mediocrity that can result when managers do not view their job as the active planning and management of the package of services being offered to physicians and patients.

Notes

An earlier version of parts of this chapter appeared as Roger Kropf and Alexander J. Szafran, "Developing a Competitive Advantage in the Market for Radiology Services," *Hospital and Health Services Administration* 33, no. 2 (Summer 1988): 213–20.

1. G. Lynn Shostack, "Service Positioning through Structural Change," in Christopher H. Lovelock, ed., *Managing Services* (Englewood Cliffs, New Jersey: Prentice-Hall, 1988), pp. 94–107.
2. Philip Kotler and Roberta N. Clarke, "Consumer Analysis," *Marketing for Health Care Organizations* (Englewood Cliffs, New Jersey: Prentice-Hall, 1987), pp. 256–288.
3. Michael E. Porter, *Competitive Advantage: Creating and Sustaining Superior Performance* (New York: Free Press, 1985), p. 36.
4. Porter, *Competitive Advantage*, p. 38.
5. Porter, *Competitive Advantage*, p. 38.
6. Porter, *Competitive Advantage*, p. 12, 14.
7. Joseph Edgar and Stephen Spearing, "Breast Imaging Center: A Total Concept," *Radiology Management*, 7, no. 2: 32–33.
8. Porter, *Competitive Advantage*, p. 70.
9. Porter, *Competitive Advantage*, p. 99.
10. T. V. Cryan, "Radiology Managers Apply Marketing," *Radiology Management* 7, no. 2 (Spring 1985): 38.

11. Porter, *Competitive Advantage*, p. 15.
12. Richard Normann, *Service Management: Strategy and Leadership in Service Businesses* (Chichester, England: John Wiley & Sons, 1984), p. 62.
13. Roger Kropf, "Competitor Analysis for Imaging Services," *Administrative Radiology* 7, no. 3 (March 1988): 41–43.
14. Kari E. Super, "Women Slow to Respond to Bone Scanning Services, While Arthritis Units Show Promise," *Modern Healthcare* (July 31, 1987): 40–42.
15. For a discussion of the theory and methods of market segmentation and research see Philip Kotler and Roberta N. Clarke, *Marketing for Health Care Organizations*.
16. Porter, *Competitive Advantage*, p. 168.
17. Normann, *Service Management*, pp. 23–24.
18. *Porter, Competitive Advantage*, p. 16.
19. Michael E. Porter and V. Millar, "How Information Gives You Competitive Advantage," *Harvard Business Review* 63, no. 4 (July–August 1985): 149–160.
20. C. Wiseman, *Strategy and Computers: Information Systems as Competitive Weapons* (Homewood, Illinois: Dow Jones–Irwin, 1985).
21. Karl Albrecht and Ron Zemke, *Service America! Doing Business in the New Economy* (Homewood, Illinois: Dow Jones–Irwin, 1985), p. 35.

Part II

The Computer Technologies and Their Benefits

4.

Service Referral and Outbound Telemarketing Systems

Description of the Technology

Hospitals, medical societies, and other organizations in many communities offer to provide consumers with a referral to a source of health care (for example, a physician or drug treatment center) or specific type of service (for example, a weight control program or blood pressure screening).

The computer technologies described in this chapter enhance this service by:

— matching the patient or physician to a provider or service using criteria they provide, or criteria suggested by a professional. (Although this can be done manually, the computer systems can provide a match using multiple criteria faster and with greater accuracy.)

— in some cases, using a nurse to make an initial assessment of need, and to advise on an appropriate course of action

— allowing the organization that operates the system to offer other services via a telephone call or through the mails, using stored telephone numbers and addresses, as well as information on an individual's characteristics, services used, and expressed needs

— permitting the organization to analyze data on the referrals requested to determine patterns (for example, volume of services used by zip code of residence), which may suggest needs that the organization could meet

Referral systems offer the capability to match a patient or physician to some group of providers by using the computer. Although most systems are designed primarily to serve potential patients, the data they store could also be helpful to physicians seeking services for their patients. *Outbound telemarketing systems* allow telephone contact (preceded or followed up with a mailing produced by a word processor) with a group of patients or physicians for the purpose of selling them a service.

Increasingly, the two types of systems are being linked and sold by the same vendor, since they both produce—and require—information on individuals who might need a service and information on the services available. Employers are also being added to the list of groups who might benefit from these systems, since employees can be provided with the information they need about available providers of care, eligibility for services, and benefits available.

Although service referral has been considered by many health care organizations as a necessary public service, calling people to offer them a service has often been considered "sales" and, therefore, too aggressive and commercial. The referral function is considered acceptable because it is passive (they call us) and impartial (the consumer is asked what they are looking for and offered a choice).

Hospitals and other organizations that have targeted specific groups of patients and physicians and are trying to actively meet their needs need to take another look at this issue, however. An organization can acquire information on patient and physician needs (1) through a phone call they make to ask for a referral, (2) through a health questionnaire or other survey, or (3) by examining bills and other records on services used. The next question is whether the organization should wait for the individual to call or make an offer to provide a service.

If patients have checked a box on a health questionnaire indicating that they want information on weight control programs, should the hospital call first or wait for them to call? Does the hospital have an obligation to offer them a competitor's program? If a hospital staff member makes the call to offer the hospital's service, is it "meeting consumer needs" or "outbound telemarketing?" While many not-for-profit organizations are committed to meeting consumer needs, outbound telemarketing is both new and, for some, unacceptably commercial.

Service Referral Systems

Description of a basic system

The simplest service referral systems operate on a personal computer with a hard disk (i.e., a device in the computer used to store large amounts of data) and use data base management software. Data base management software allows the user to select one or more data items (for example, a zip code, age) and ask for any stored data that match it. The user might, for example, ask for any gynecologists between 35 and 50 whose office is in zip code 10003. The computer will list all the physicians (for whom information is available) who meet these criteria.

One or a hundred characteristics of a physician could be stored, depending on how much effort and money the organization wishes to expend on collecting and updating the desired data. The system can easily be expanded to provide information on services such as drug treatment.

Enhancements

Enhancements to the basic system just described include:

— a *network version* that allows more than one person to use the system. Special software is required to link more than one personal computer (or several terminals) to a single personal computer (i.e., a "file server") that contains the data and software for referrals.

— a *word processor* that uses patient addresses and other data stored to produce correspondence (for example, a letter to the physician saying that a referral has been made). Software must be included that carries out the transfer of the necessary data. The word-processing software may also be customized to allow the storage of letters, which can be automatically produced by selecting an item on the screen from a "menu" (i.e., a list of available options). A letter-quality printer is, of course, required.

— *medical protocols* that allow the user to enter symptoms, problems, and complaints and to retrieve advice on the options available to the patient. A caller may have received a blow to the head and have a headache. The medical protocol might ask if the patient has been vomiting and advise a visit to the emergency room.

— *spreadsheet, statistical, graphics, and mapping software* that allows for the aggregation of data in the computer, the preparation of means, medians, and other statistics, charts and graphs, and maps showing information such as what percentage of callers reside in various zip codes or towns. The vendor may not provide this software, but instead provide software that helps in moving the required data to such programs, which the organization purchases itself.

— *the ability to do patient and class scheduling.* While basic systems require that the operator put the patient on hold and telephone a physician's office to make an appointment (some systems facilitate

this with automatic dialing), the system itself can include a scheduler that allows the operator to make the appointment directly.
Systems can also include the scheduling of weight loss and other
classes, and maintain rosters for them.

— a *program for admission reconciliation.* If data on inpatient admissions or outpatient visits are entered, a program in the system
matches records on callers, allowing the identification of patients
who actually received a service. The additional revenue received
can then be identified.[1]

Outbound Telemarketing Systems

Description of a basic system

Outbound telemarketing systems can be purchased alone, or in combination
with service referral systems. A simple outbound telemarketing system purchased alone would include a personal computer with a hard disk and data
base management software that allows for the storage and retrieval of data on
potential customers. A list of potential customers is obtained in some manner,
and the individuals are called. Data are then entered, including the person's
name and address, when contact was made, the result, and further action to
be taken.

Enhancements

Enhancements that are available include:

— stored *scripts* that provide either word-for-word text of what should
be said or reminders to the operator to touch on certain points.

— support for *membership management* programs (for example, senior citizen, maternity). The special software allows the user to process new member applications, respond to requests for information,
produce direct mail campaigns, and track member purchases and
revenues generated.

— *software and data to actually register* a person for a program or
service. This requires that a schedule be maintained. The alternative
is to indicate that the person will receive a call later.

— *software that links the system to a service referral system* so that
both use the same data bases.

— *power-dialing*, so that the computer can be told to dial a group of
telephone numbers until someone answers, and then to display
information on the individual who has been called. This increases
the efficiency of the process since a person does not have to be paid
to dial the phone number and wait for an answer. It also means that

data are readily available, including services that the individual has expressed an interest in.

— *word-processing* software with the capability to generate correspondence easily (as described earlier).

The "Purchase or Develop" Decision

The computer hardware and software for creating a service referral or outbound telemarketing system could be purchased at any computer store from components that are used for many other purposes. This would include a computer, a hard disk, and a general-purpose data base management program. A more advanced system could also be assembled to provide some of the functions that will be discussed in this chapter. The issue is whether a health care organization has the staff, money, or both to customize the system to do exactly what it wants.

For example, what the user of the system sees on the screen when they turn it on, and what they have to do to retrieve data, can be very easy for someone with little computer expertise to handle, or may require hours of training. The difference is the amount of time that has been spent by a professional customizing the system to make it unnecessary for the user to do more than follow simple instructions.

A vendor who has developed a system can offer the user an easy-to-use product, assistance in collecting and entering the data needed, training, updates that reflect advances in software, further customization, and help in restoring the system if there is a hardware or software failure.

The market for basic systems has become very competitive; prices for the software for a physician referral system alone can be as low as $5,500 (with no training or maintenance included). Given the salaries and consulting fees of computer programmers, health care organizations should carefully examine any proposal to develop such a system internally to determine if the full costs have been accurately and completely estimated (which is very difficult to do). Health care organizations that hire an additional employee to manage a referral or outbound telemarketing system will incur, of course, labor costs that may be substantially higher than the cost of the hardware and software. This is true even if a complete system is purchased from a vendor.

Potential for Enhancing Services

Communicating with and Serving Potential Customers

Once a target market has been identified and the hospital, physician group, or other provider is prepared to deliver excellent services, communication with the targeted patients and physicians is essential.

Referral systems

Referral systems can be used to communicate the availability of services. An offer can be made through various media, including direct mail, to potential patients and physicians to use the referral system. The computer can then be used to match patients and physicians with the physicians and services they feel are appropriate, using many criteria including the type of specialty, office location, hours, and method of payment. The speed with which a patient can be matched is also increased when compared with published sources that are often out-of-date or lack information important to individual patients.

Since the computer stores the name, telephone number, patient problem, and the referral made, improved follow-up and problem resolution are possible. Patients can be called to ask about their progress and their satisfaction with services. Personal attention from friendly staff during the initial call and any follow-up can enhance perceptions that the organization cares.

The flow of information to physicians can be improved when referral systems have word-processing capabilities that provide for automatic correspondence to the physician who has received a referral. Physicians' practices are also supported through increased referrals.

Outbound telemarketing systems

The benefits of outbound telemarketing systems to the patient or physician include improved access to a service or physician because of the information received, and a better match of consumers with providers (i.e., each finds the other desirable on the basis of their objectives and preferences). As a result of personal attention from friendly staff, there may also be an enhanced perception that the sponsoring organization cares about patients and can provide individualized services. An organization that follows up a health awareness campaign with an offer to provide information or a referral to an individual with an identified health risk is likely to be viewed as more professional. One system calls patients (at their request) to remind them to refill their prescriptions at a local pharmacy. The computer automatically dials the numbers and leaves a prerecorded message.[2]

The system also allows for resolving problems that may be faced by patients seeking services. Patients who were registered for a service can also be called back later to determine if the organization can help in resolving any further problems the patient faces (for example, transportation).

As with referral systems, the flow of information to physicians can be improved when telemarketing systems have word-processing capabilities that provide for automatic correspondence to the physician who has received a referral. Physicians' practices are also supported through increased referrals.

The Employer and Third-Party Payer as Customer

A referral system can be used to provide information on benefits and the available service network to hospitals and physicians who serve the members of various HMOs, PPOs, and insurance plans, relieving the employer or third-party payer of some of the burden of providing this information.

Examples

The Inter+Net Health Systems case in Part IV provides a detailed description of the steps required in implementing a physician and service referral system. The examples in this section are provided only as illustrations of some of the capabilities of systems on the market in 1990, and of how vendors describe the payoffs that might be achieved.

Referral Systems

Appendix A is an excerpt from the marketing literature for Referral One and Service Referral One, products of National Health Enhancement Systems, Inc., of Phoenix, Arizona. They require the basic hardware described earlier.

Outbound Telemarketing Systems

Appendix B provides a description of the outbound telemarketing system that is also offered by National Health Enhancement Systems, Inc., of Phoenix, Arizona. It requires the basic hardware described earlier with at least a 30 MB (megabytes), as opposed to a 20 MB, hard disk drive.

Appendix C describes the Central Contact System[SM] offered by LVM Systems of Tempe, Arizona. The Central Contact System is an attempt to centralize the management of an organization's contacts with a wide variety of markets, including employers and industry. It provides a means of tracking those contacts, and scheduling future contacts to assure that they are made.

The Financial Payoff

The calls that Georgetown University Hospital in Washington fielded in a six-month period (October 1987 to March 1988) of operating its "Georgetown M.D." referral service resulted in $1.1 million in revenue. The 3,302 referrals made during that period resulted in 120 inpatient admissions, 58 same-day surgeries, and 69 emergency room visits. In addition, callers used various ancillary services 694 times.[3] Georgetown used PhysicianLine software by HealthLine Systems of San Diego, California.

At Scripps Memorial Hospital in La Jolla, California, each referral made by its "HealthCare Finder" service generated $400–$500 in revenue.[4] Scripps jointly developed the software with the firm of Arthur Young of Los Angeles, California.

Tables 14.1 and 14.2 of the Inter+Net case in Part IV (Chapter 14) show the projected demand, revenue, and profitability in year one for Inter+Net's Ask-A-Nurse® physician and service referral system (Ask-A-Nurse is a registered trademark of Referral Systems Group, Inc., Citrus Heights, California). Ask-A-Nurse uses software by both Referral Systems Group in Roseville, California, and Baxter Healthcare Corporation in Deerfield, Illinois.

Appendix B shows the financial impact of an "exemplary" program of screening 10,000 patients for cancer and/or heart disease. National Health Enhancement Systems (NHES) projects that a hospital could expect gross, direct referral revenue of $662,250 and a net contribution to fixed costs and profit of $297,000 during the first year. This excludes the cost of purchasing a franchise from NHES.

Both Appendix B and the projections in the Inter+Net case make a number of assumptions that may or may not be reasonable for a specific hospital. The usefulness of this type of analysis, which uses assumptions rather than historical hospital and market area data, is to allow a decision maker to prepare a financial forecast before a program is begun. The forecast can be based on assumptions, and then those assumptions can be changed to test how sensitive the results are to any particular one.

As NHES notes, the results in Appendix B could be achieved by an "exemplary" program. In order to achieve these results, the staff resources must be available to conduct the screening of 10,000 people and to make a follow-up contact with 3,500 of them. NHES includes only incremental costs and assumes that an infrastructure, including office space, telephone, and secretarial support, is available at no cost to support the program.

The hospital must also have the clinical resources to deliver care to the numbers of people shown in Appendix B, Exhibit D3. All of this activity must be completed in 12 months to get the annual revenue indicated. Fees must be close to those indicated, and marginal costs for direct patient care must be 50 percent of gross direct referral revenue (minus incremental direct operating costs).

Alternative assumptions could be tested to determine their projected financial impact. If the incidence of health problems is known to be lower than the estimates in Appendix B, Exhibit D1, for example, the number of people who would be contacted could be reduced from 3,500 to a lower figure, resulting in a reduction in profits and contribution to fixed costs. If labor costs are higher, or the productivity of current workers suggest that additional workers will be needed, then labor costs could be increased.

Health care organizations considering the acquisition of a service referral system or outbound telemarketing system need to prepare such forecasts and engage decision makers and the vendor in a discussion of what assumptions must be true to achieve the desired results.

Selecting the Components of a System

In this chapter, the extent to which various computer systems have been linked to provide an active rather than passive system for managing contacts with patient, physicians, and employers has been described to make some of the options clear. A referral system can be purchased alone, or as part of a system that includes outbound telemarketing and the capability to keep track of contacts made with a variety of the organization's customers, including the medical staff, members of a club for senior citizens, and actual and potential donors.

Vendors appear now to see their role as assisting in the management of communications with a wide variety of markets. Although the markets were initially defined as potential patients, physicians and employers have now been added to the list. These systems were initially somewhat simple applications of data base management software; they have been enhanced by adding other types of programs that help in mailing and telephoning, in managing staff time, and in evaluation.

The new systems assume that a very active staff is in contact regularly with its potential customers and is continually evaluating the success of the organization's programs. Organizations that have (or want) this intense level of activity are likely to find one of these products attractive; organizations without a service strategy or active marketing program will find it difficult to justify the cost.

Notes

1. David Albachten, "Proving Return on Investment: Computerized Tracking and Admissions Reconciliation," *Computers in Healthcare* 10, no. 1 (January 1989): 30–36.
2. "Computer Reminder Improves Compliance: Med-Minder Calls Patients When Their Prescriptions Need Refilling," *Chain Store Age Executive* 65 (April 1989): 67–68.
3. Michele von Dambrowski, *Physician Referral Services* (Rye, New York: Health Care Communications, 1988), p. 73.
4. Von Dambrowski, *Physician Referral Services,* p. 9.

5.

Scheduling and Tracking Systems

Description of the Technology

Most health care organizations offer some or all of their services to patients who have previously been scheduled. Schedules are often maintained in one or more books. Although this simple arrangement can work effectively, computer systems offer a number of benefits:

— They allow clerical staff to make many changes without reducing the legibility of the appointment schedule, a frequent occurrence as appointments in pencil are changed, as more patients are added, and as the availability of a physician or other provider changes.

— They have the ability to notice and report on conflicts, such as the unavailability of a resource (for example, a CT scanner) at a time when a patient has been scheduled to receive a service.

— They have the ability to prompt staff to investigate the need for the requested (or additional) procedures. Some systems report if the requested procedure (or an alternative, similar procedure) has recently been performed on the patient, or if additional procedures are required with the requested procedure.

— They can be linked with other management systems (for example, by sharing a common data base) so that necessary tasks are not left undone. The system may even execute some tasks automatically without clerical staff reentering data. The scheduling system could, for example, not only cause a notice to be sent to medical records on a particular day to have a patient's medical chart sent to a clinic, but also create a "pull list" (a list of charts to be pulled from storage) that prints out in the medical records department.

— They can provide reports, including tables and graphs, that provide management with a picture of what is happening in the organization and how it differs from desired standards.

Since a scheduling system is often the first management system to receive information on a patient or physician who wishes to utilize a service, it can be used to provide data to a system that subsequently tracks what later happens.

Manual tracking systems are also used by many health care organizations. Such systems include the patient record and bill, employee records showing time worked, and schedules for the use of particular rooms or pieces of equipment. Computer systems offer a number of benefits:

— Legibility.

— The ability to be linked to other management systems, as noted earlier.

— The ability to track the location of the patient, beginning with registration. The time the patient has spent in each stage of receiving the services (for example, in the waiting room, in an exam room) can be monitored so that managers can take whatever actions are needed to minimize waiting time.

— The ability to note where gaps and inaccuracies in the data might exist. For example, the system can report to a manager when an appointment was made and kept, but when the tasks required by other systems (for example, the creation of a bill) were not carried out.

— The ability to produce management reports.

Although this description has suggested that scheduling and tracking are two separate systems, they are now commonly linked.

Other vendors offer separate products, however, and the implementation of a tracking system involves the training of a larger number of staff than those who carry out the scheduling function. If a tracking system that uses bar coding is desired, special hardware is also required. Bar codes are the series of lines, now found on most packaged goods, that can be quickly read by a device called a scanner, which enters the data into the computer. Because of the differences in the staff used and hardware required, the two systems will be discussed separately.

Scheduling Systems

Description of a basic system

The simplest scheduling systems operate on a personal computer with a hard disk (i.e., a device in the computer used to store large amounts of data) and use software that creates a data base that includes data on the dates and times services are available, and the individuals who are scheduled to provide and use the services. A scheduling system could be created using data base management software that had the ability to present the data as a series of reports (for example, patients scheduled by day and hour of the week for a specific physician).

Enhancements

Enhancements to the basic system just described could include the following:

— The ability to check for many types of conflicts using rules supplied by management. For example, the system could check the availability of a microscope for surgery when someone attempts to schedule a patient for surgery that requires one.

— A link to the organization's central computer to avoid having to enter data already stored and to allow for the updating of the other data bases in the organization (for example, accounting and billing).

— A word processor that allows for the production of reports, lists, labels for the organization, and customized forms and letters for the patient and referring physician. The production of these items could be made automatic, or an item could be prepared and sent at the request of the operator. A letter-quality printer would be required for correspondence.

— A report generator, that is, software that produces tables, statistics, and graphs. Instead of providing this software, the vendor may provide software that helps in moving the required data to such programs, which the organization purchases itself.

— A network version that allows more than one person to use the system. Special software is required to link more than one personal computer (or several terminals) to a single personal computer (i.e., a "file server") that contains the data and software for scheduling. If the organization uses several sites but wishes to maintain a single scheduling system, telecommunications hardware and software could also be provided.

— Software that allows a physician's office or a facility to use the scheduling system from a remote site, using telephone lines and a modem for communication.

Tracking Systems

Description of a basic system

The simplest tracking systems also operate on a personal computer with a hard disk and use software that creates one or more data bases. Data could be stored on:

1. the use of resources such as operating rooms and supplies
2. staff time and activity
3. the movement of the patient through the process of receiving the service

Such a system could again be created using data base management software that had the ability to present the data as a series of reports.

Enhancements

Enhancements to the basic system could include the following:

— The hardware and software to produce and read bar-coded labels.

— A word processor that allows for the automatic insertion of data collected in a variety of documents, including reports of the results of a procedure.

— A link to the organization's central computer to allow for the exchange of data with other systems, for example, billing.

— A report generator or software that allows data to be sent to where management reports can be produced.

— A network version that allows more than one person to use the system. Special software is required to link more than one personal computer (or several terminals) to a single personal computer (i.e., a "file server") that contains the necessary data and software.

Bar coding

Bar codes are a series of vertical lines that can be read by a special device called a scanner.[1] The scanner looks like a pencil or a handgun and is used to point ordinary light or a laser beam at the bar code. The lines produce a pattern that is transmitted to a computer, which compares this pattern with others stored in the computer to identify what the bar code means. In a supermarket, each product is assigned a code, which is turned into a bar code that can be read by the computer.

Bar codes have multiple uses in a health care organization.[2] The bar code could be used in exactly the same way to identify medical supplies. When a nurse or clerk removes supplies from a supply cabinet, for example, the bar code on the items could be read by a scanner. Management would then know what supplies had been removed and could decide how many units to order.

Bar codes could also be used to identify people. Some tracking systems produce a bar code for each person scheduled to receive a service and print the bar code on peel-off labels and/or an inpatient's wristband.[3] The labels can be removed and put on patient registration forms, order slips, film jackets, specimen bottles, and any other object or form that is associated with the care of the patient.

When a blood test is ordered, for example, a bar code for that individual can be placed on both the order form and the specimen bottle. When the blood is drawn, the nurse or clerk can use a scanner to enter the patient's code into the computer. When the lab receives the specimen bottle, the lab tech would use a scanner to enter the patient's code. Parkland Memorial Hospital in Dallas has attached a bar code reader to a blood analyzer, allowing the analyzer itself to transmit the results to the laboratory's management information system, where they are available almost immediately for review.[4] The bar codes allow managers to track blood samples by having the computer compare all those patients whose blood has been drawn with those whose samples have been tested.

Bar coding requires the purchase of software to create and read the bar codes, hardware to produce the bar-coded labels, and scanners to read the codes. Additional terminals or personal computers may also be needed. Most scanners are attached by a cable to a terminal or personal computer. Portable scanners are available that store information for later transmission to a terminal or personal computer through another special piece of hardware.

The "Purchase or Develop" Decision

The issues here are similar to those described in Chapter 4. The computer hardware and software for creating a scheduling and tracking system could be purchased at any computer store from components that are used for many other purposes. This would include a computer, a hard disk and a general-purpose data base management program. A more advanced system could also be assembled to provide some of the functions that are discussed in this chapter. The issue is whether a health care organization has the staff, money, or both to customize the system to do exactly what it wants.

Bar coding technology, in particular, may raise problems. Although it is commonly used in large-scale systems developed by supermarket chains and banks, expertise on its use for health care applications may be scarce in many communities. The use of bar code hardware that is not serviced by a local retailer may also lead to problems, especially when the system is integrated into clinical systems where the expectation by physicians and others is that a failure, if one occurs, will be very rapidly corrected.

Aside from bar coding, a major question that needs to be faced is the trade-off between ease-of-use and the cost of development. For example, how easy it is to use the system will depend on the amount of time that has been spent by a professional customizing the system.

A vendor who has developed a system can offer the user an easy-to-use product, assistance in collecting and entering the data needed, training, updates that reflect advances in software, further customization, and help in restoring the system if there is a hardware or software failure.

Managers need to compare the cost of a system to the estimated cost of development. Health care organizations should carefully examine any proposal to develop a system internally to determine if the full costs have been accurately and completely estimated. Software development projects often require more time than was initially estimated, however, since the needs of users often become clear only after they review a test system. Systems analysts and programmers also have difficulty estimating the number of hours that will be required for design and programming, which is creative work.

Potential for Enhancing Services

Scheduling Systems

Scheduling systems can reduce errors by checking if the necessary resources are available (for example, physicians and equipment) and by checking that the scheduled procedure is not equivalent to one already performed or is not inappropriate for a variety of reasons. Patient perceptions of competence can be improved by providing patients with customized information (via a computer link or through a word processor and the mails) on topics such as how to reach the facility or preparations for a procedure. Scheduling systems can also track each person and procedure to assist in follow-up and problem resolution.

Because the availability of resources can be checked, scheduling systems can provide more flexible scheduling to accommodate patients' personal needs (for example, a family vacation).

Scheduling systems can be combined with a link or word-processing system that generates correspondence to improve the flow of information to the referring physician, for example, concerning when a test has been scheduled or when the results will be ready.

Tracking Systems

Tracking systems can improve a manager's control of the process of providing health services. Reports can be prepared on the time needed to perform a task (for example, registering a patient or doing a chest x-ray) and the resources used, offering the possibility of reducing waiting time and, therefore, the speed with which the service is provided. Because the patient's identity, procedure, time, location, and staff involved in rendering a service are recorded, follow-up and problem resolution can be improved.

Such systems also allow for the control of inventory to assure that items are available when they are needed. The location of films and medical records can also be tracked in this way. A referring physician could benefit from improved access to information, such as medical records and images, that results from more accurate tracking of their location.

Example

Appendix D is an excerpt from the marketing literature for the Operating Room Scheduling Office System (ORSOS) by the Atwork Corporation of San Jose, California.

The Financial Payoff

The financial impact of improved patient and physician satisfaction with services is difficult to quantify. No studies of the impact of scheduling and tracking systems on patient or physician use were uncovered in preparing this chapter.

Vendors tend to justify the costs of these systems by suggesting that improvements in charge capture (i.e., the number of charges for services received that are actually included on the patient's bill), enhanced staff productivity, lower inventory costs, and improved throughput will more than pay the costs.

A health care organization trying to decide whether to make a purchase might begin by looking at the issue of lost charges by sampling current services/procedures/visits to determine what proportion of the resources actually used were entered into the accounting system. The number of duplicative tests performed may also be used to examine the issue of whether tighter controls would yield significant savings.

Where resources are being used at close to capacity, the issue of whether throughput (the number of services per hour or day) could be improved might then be examined. Techniques for examining the issue of throughput and the possible improvements that might be gained by carefully monitoring the process are well developed and routinely applied in some health care organizations.[5]

The potential for improvements in staff productivity are harder to assess. Minimum staffing needs may prevent reductions in staffing; health care organizations that cannot obtain enough staff to fill vacant positions will need to estimate the opportunity costs (i.e., the money that would otherwise be spent if staff were available) rather than actual cash savings. The impact of being able to provide more services with less work on the morale of overworked staff could be substantial, but again is difficult to quantify.

This discussion is not meant to suggest that the financial benefits of using these systems is likely to be small. Anecdotal evidence suggests that the volume of lost charges, the cost of unbillable duplicative services, and the lost revenue when resources are not fully utilized are very large in some health care organizations. Often lacking is a system for continuous monitoring of the size of the existing problem and any improvement. Paradoxically, these computer systems are useful in carrying out this monitoring and evaluating function but must be purchased before the information can become available to justify purchasing them.

Organizations committed to service excellence may wish to justify a purchase on the basis of enhanced satisfaction measured through surveys and other methods. What is clearly needed, however, are studies that demonstrate that such improvements in satisfaction lead to higher service volume (and additional net revenues) by more satisfied patients and physicians. Organizations that purchase these systems should make the inclusion of a system for monitoring and evaluating service volume (or software to move data to where such an evaluation will be performed) a major criterion in deciding on which system to purchase.

Selecting the Components of a System

There are many reasons why a health care organization should consider acquiring a system that allows for both scheduling and tracking. The advantages of linking the two systems have already been discussed. By linking the two systems, a health care organization gains the ability to treat the patient's encounter with the organization as a single continuous process from the initial request for an appointment to a final billing.

As has already been pointed out, however, the two systems require different resources. The organization considering both needs to decide whether it has the internal capabilities to implement them.

Scheduling systems are used by clerical staff, but tracking systems will have to be used by many more people. A tracking system that requires that physicians and technologists run a scanner over a bar code label assumes that compliance with this procedure will be consistent and automatic. As Mari Malvey has documented in her study of the implementation of a hospital financial information system, such compliance should not be assumed.[6] Planning, the involvement of a wide range of staff, and careful thinking about how to motivate people to support a system are needed. Tracking systems will also require that hardware such as terminals and bar code readers be available where people work in sufficient quantity to assure that limited access does not result in reduced compliance.

Health care organizations may wish to acquire a system with the capabilities to do both scheduling and tracking, and implement each component as it becomes clear that the resources are available and that compliance by staff with the new procedures is likely.

Notes

1. Craig Harmon and Russ Adams, *Reading between the Lines: An Introduction to Bar Code Technology* (Peterborough, New Hampshire: Helmers Publishing, 1984).
2. American Hospital Association, *Bar Code Technology—Applications in Health Care* (Chicago: American Hospital Publishing, 1984).
3. Michael Maffetone, Suzanne Watt, and Kenneth Whisler, "Automated Sample Handling in a Clinical Laboratory," *Computers in Health Care* 9, no. 11 (1988): 48–50.
4. Susan Steane and Debra Hale, "Bar Code Earns Respect," *Computers in Health Care* 9, no. 11 (1988): 52–54.
5. D. Michael Warner, Don C. Holloway, and Kyle L. Grazier, *Decision Making and Control for Health Administration, second edition* (Ann Arbor, Michigan: Health Administration Press, 1984).
6. Mari Malvey, *Simple Systems, Complex Environments: Hospital Financial Information Systems* (Beverly Hills, California: Sage Publications, 1981).

6.

Market Analysis Systems

Description of the Technology

Market analysis systems are the direct result of the revolution in personal computing that has occurred during the 1970s and 1980s. All of the features offered by current systems were available separately on mainframe computers in the early 1970s, but the user was required to purchase or obtain a license to use a number of separate programs for the mainframe. The cost of a license for a single statistical program might be thousands of dollars per year. Consequently, only the employees or students in a university or large corporation had access to the statistical, modeling, mapping, and graphics programs now available on a personal computer.

The personal computers available in the 1970s did not, however, have the memory needed to link all four types of programs so that a user could move from producing a table to a graph to a map with a few keystrokes. The large-capacity, fast hard disk drives for personal computers that became available during the 1980s were needed.

Vendors are now offering systems that have the capability to perform statistical analyses, to test assumptions by changing numbers and observing the changes in related variables (i.e., modeling), and then to graph or map the results. Not only can the user move from one task to another with a few keystrokes, but changes in a number of related tables, maps, and graphs might occur automatically as individual data or assumptions are changed. The hardware required costs from $3,000 (for a personal computer with a color monitor and hard disk), to $5,000–10,000 for an advanced personal computer (using a fast "386" memory chip, and as much internal and hard disk memory as a minicomputer), to more than $20,000 for a minicomputer that would be fully compatible with the computer being used in a hospital's central data-processing system.

In looking at the benefits of purchasing a system, the comparison that needs to be made is between assembling a system from hardware available in a computer store to purchasing a system that is ready to operate. The benefits of a ready-to-operate system from a vendor are the following:

— Software is provided that links the various software packages so that data are moved automatically from one to the other (for example, from a modeling program to a mapping program). Although "integrated" programs can be purchased in a computer store that link a modeling program (for example, a spreadsheet) to a graphics and data base management program, none of them now include the capability to prepare maps.

— The software and data bases supplied can be highly customized to fit the needs of health care organizations. Although a spreadsheet program available in a computer store could produce an estimate of revenue from a new service if the appropriate formulas and data were entered, a customized product provided for the health care industry could include alternative formulas for projection and the specific facility data required. The more customized the product, however, the higher the cost.

— In particular, the vendor can develop data bases, that is, assemble the data required and put them in a form that can be immediately used by the system. Vendors offer services that range from instructions on how to prepare the necessary data bases to telephone assistance to on-site assistance. Prices vary dramatically, of course.

— The vendor can also provide services that enhance what the system can do. These services can range from the development of specialized data bases from external sources (for example, data on hospital use at specific competing hospitals) to the preparation of customized reports. Organizations can then decide whether to do a task internally or pay to have it done by the vendor.

— The vendor can offer training by individuals who have worked with other health care organizations. A local consultant may have little experience in working with data on health services or on the problems being analyzed. An organization that develops its own system can face a crisis when a staff member who developed the system leaves without preparing adequate documentation. Vendors can provide a pool of knowledgeable staff and systems documentation.

Description of a Basic System

A basic system consists of a personal computer with a hard disk, a color monitor, and a letter-quality printer. Software that can manage data bases (i.e., store data and permit the quick retrieval of the data), produce tabular reports, calculate statistics, create and run models, produce graphics, and create maps is included. A basic system would come with instructions on how to create the necessary data bases. Only simple models that use generic techniques would be included, rather than complex models that attempt to simulate how patients and physicians behave in the health care industry.

Enhancements

Enhancements to the basic system could include the following:

— A *color plotter* to allow for the production of color graphs and maps without sending a diskette to an outside service (with a delay of 24 hours or more).

— Hardware for *backing up the data* in the system easily. The alternative is to use diskettes, which can be a lengthy process. If staff fail to frequently back up the data, a failure in the system could result in the loss of data that cost thousands of dollars of staff time to produce.

— *Customized data bases* of both internal and external data. Vendor staff can provide services that range from entering data from sheets provided by the organization to on-site assistance and quality checking. Census and other data for a specific community can be selected and put into the buyer's computer.

— *Models* that are specific both to the buyer and the environment. A vendor can prepare a model that projects additional revenue from a new service in the same way it has been done manually by an organization, or even work to create an acceptable model where none has existed. A model that attempts to project revenue based on state-specific reimbursement rules could also be provided.

— The system can be *linked* to other systems in the organization, such as an accounting system, to assure that the most current data are always used. The link could be a program that the user must run to exchange data. The computer that is used to operate the market analysis system could also be networked with other computers so that data could be more easily shared.

— The system can be highly *integrated.* All the software and data bases could then be used by operators without their having to move data from one software program to another, and without having to update a data base when a change is made (for example, a new assumption about charges is added). The user must learn only one set of commands (for example, to print a report) regardless of what task was being performed. Integration is not really an enhancement to a system, but a characteristic of the system itself. It should be a major factor in deciding which system to purchase.

The "Purchase or Develop" Decision

Since software and hardware to perform all the functions of a basic system are available from computer stores, many organizations will ask why they need to pay the higher price charged by a vendor. In fact, vendors recognize this issue by providing hardware specifications and offering to support a variety of different hardware made by various manufacturers.

The major issue is who provides the software and data bases. Staff competence, cost, and the time frame of the buyer are factors. Some organizations have no staff with the skills needed to combine generic software into a system. Other organizations have competent staff, but the cost involved in creating a system from scratch would be greater than purchasing a vendor's product.

The most difficult situation exists when an organization with an active marketing and planning staff has already created data bases and acquired or developed software that performs many of the functions that have been described. The issue here is likely to be integration, that is, it is time consuming to prepare the tables, statistics, maps, and graphs that managers often ask for with little notice. A highly integrated system would allow the job to be done faster and might also allow managers to do some of the work themselves, without relying on computer professionals or planning and marketing staff with advanced skills.

The "buy vs. develop" decision is complex (and the replacement decision even more so). Managers should, at a minimum, evaluate the capabilities of systems on the market periodically to keep aware of the capabilities that have been developed. A discussion with organizations that use a system is very important, and vendors are glad to supply the names of satisfied customers.

Managers should be especially cautious about deciding to develop a system from scratch internally. The costs of developing a system are difficult to estimate precisely unless only a minimum of customization is desired. If management is simply interested in taking advantage of the capabilities of available programs (as may have already occurred in finance and other areas), the expense of a specialized system from a vendor may not be justified.

Managers should, however, be cautious about approving the development of systems that are expected to provide sophisticated modeling capabilities using local data bases that the organization has little experience in using. There are two heavy prices the organization could pay. The first is higher-than-expected costs for a system that never meets the original specifications. The second is the cost of making poor decisions because a system that looked like it was working was, in fact, providing incorrect information.

Asking a vendor to produce a highly customized system can also be risky, but the buyer has the opportunity to ask for a demonstration of a similar system that worked and talk to other health care organizations that have relied on it.

The critical issue for health care organizations is whether they are willing to devote one or more staff with sufficient ability, interest, and free time to master the software and hardware, regardless of whether it is provided by the vendor or assembled internally. Although staff may be able to produce a few reports after a short training session, using market analysis systems to their full potential is not a quick or easy process. Staff who use such systems intermittently will not gain the proficiency to produce complex reports that exploit the data bases that are currently available. Assigning a single junior staff member to learn the system while performing other duties does not respond to the problem; they are generally unaware of what managers need to know, while more senior managers remain unfamiliar with what the new system is capable of producing. There is generally no substitute for assigning at least one experienced manager with an interest in learning the task of using the system, and providing that person with the time to do it.

Potential for Enhancing Services

Market analysis systems can reduce the staff time and skill required to retrieve, analyze, and produce the tables, maps, and graphs needed to define a market based on where patients and physicians live, their prior use of health services, and demographic and economic characteristics such as age, family size, and income. When financial models are included, the staff time and skill needed to estimate demand, and assess the profitability of providing services to these markets, are also reduced.

This can result in improved access to services for these targeted patients and physicians. By carefully identifying the characteristics of the markets it wishes to serve, an organization is able to design services that better match the needs and preferences of these patients and physicians, increasing their satisfaction with services.

Support can be provided to referring physicians by providing them with market analyses that could be useful in targeting groups they wish to serve.

Examples

The examples in this section are provided only as illustrations of some of the capabilities of systems on the market in 1990, and of how vendors describe the payoffs that might result.

Two Market Analysis Systems

Appendixes E and F are brief descriptions of The Market Planner® and its extension, the Physician Practice Planner™, products of the Sachs Group of Evanston, Illinois. A brief description of the Marketing Systems Library is given in Appendix G. This software is a product of the Decision Support Services Division of HBO & Company of Atlanta, Georgia.

A Case Study

Appendix H is a case study prepared jointly by HBO & Company and MediQual Systems, Inc., of Westborough, Massachusetts, using the Marketing Systems Library (with data produced by HBO's Case Mix Library software and Clinical Cost Accounting Systems) and MediQual's Medical Illness Severity Groupings Systems (MedisGroups) software. Robert Bradbury and Frank Stearns, Jr., have described some of the possible uses of the Medis-Groups system, which both defines clinical severity and identifies cases where clinical evidence provides little support for a course of treatment.[1]

In this case, existing demographic trends and information on current market share were examined to determine the potential demand for obstetrical services by members of an HMO. Internal data were then examined to determine whether it might be possible to reduce the number of C-sections being performed. The financial implications of a reduction in the number of C-sections and an increase in patient volume were then examined.

This case illustrates the potential of market analysis systems to be expanded through linkages with other computer systems to become "decision support systems" for a wide variety of decisions in a health care organization. A decision support system is a computer-based system for storing and analyzing data to assist the leadership of an organization in making decisions. Earlier decision support systems offered access to fewer data bases and had much more limited capability to display easily the information in a variety of ways (for example, tables, maps, and graphs).[2]

The Financial Payoff

As the case study in Appendix H suggests, the payoff from a market analysis system could be very large. It is important to note, however, that market analysis systems do not generate revenue themselves. Whether any revenue is obtained depends on the success of the activity being undertaken. A change in state reimbursement, the failure of staff to properly implement the program, and other factors could result in no revenue being received.

The systems are also passive tools. In the hands of a skilled manager, they can lead to decisions that enhance revenue. In the hands of a manager unable to develop and implement new programs, or make changes in existing ones, they could result in no additional revenue.

It is also important to consider the effect of the capabilities of these systems on decision makers. If management relies on intuition or successful models elsewhere in deciding to implement a program, the market analysis system (and market analysis) is redundant.

When decision makers want better information, when opportunities are available and the organization has the capability to respond to them, and when failure is a real possibility because of competition and other factors— then a market analysis system could have a major payoff for an organization.

Selecting the Components of a System

In selecting components, it is important to distinguish between hardware options, applications software, and data bases. A color plotter could be added, and a back-up system purchased. The issue is the time that it takes to produce the same results without these enhancements. Managers need to ask their staffs to estimate the costs of alternatives and the time involved, and to determine if an in-house capability is necessary. For example, a continual flow of requests by the board or senior management for analyses supported by graphics make a color plotter highly desirable.

The software options purchased will depend on the volume of activity in the specific area involved. For example, the Physician Practice Planner is an add-on being offered by the Sachs Group to deal with a specific topic— physicians. The volume of activity and priority given to this area will determine its desirability. Managers should be careful to determine that the add-on product is fully integrated with the main system and/or to calculate the costs involved in installing and operating it. A system that requires learning a new set of commands or the development of a major new data base could generate much higher costs than the price of the software itself.

Data bases are likely to present the major dilemma for an organization selecting a system. A statement such as "data on product costs are required" does not begin to reflect the large problems involved in creating a high-quality data base in this area. A high-quality data base on product costs may not be possible in an organization without a major change in the accounting and clinical information systems of the organization, at a cost that could run into millions of dollars. It depends on the quality of the existing information systems. Before management commits itself to a product because of its sophisticated and attractive capabilities, the cost of providing the data bases that are required must be estimated. A simpler system with fewer capabilities may be more consistent with the quantity and quality of the data currently available.

The amount of external data that the organization should purchase is another major question. Data from the census are available at a relatively low cost, but proprietary data bases on consumer purchasing patterns may carry a much higher price tag. Some vendors require that a fee be paid every time such data are requested. Data on costs in competing hospitals may come with the system, but since such data are collected annually, the acquisition of the data becomes a recurring cost.

Which data bases are purchased should depend on a projection of the types of decisions that are likely to be made. Detailed consumer purchasing data and demographics on all zip codes may be unnecessary, while demographic data for cities and towns could be made a regular purchase (every two to five years depending on the source).

The dilemma in purchasing any computer-based tool for analysis—from a spreadsheet program to data bases—is how to balance the initial attractiveness of a capability with the real needs of the organization's decision makers. Continual feedback of the information to those decision makers and observation of what information they use in conversation and in writing is one suggested process for decision making. Charts and graphs that are never quoted, presented, or in any way referred to may represent a luxury that many health care organizations cannot afford.

Notes

1. Robert C. Bradbury and Frank E. Stearns, Jr., "Managing Hospital Quality through a Clinical Severity Approach," *Journal of Health Care Marketing* 9, no. 2 (June 1989): 13–19.
2. Roger Kropf and James A. Greenberg, "Developing a Decision Support System," *Strategic Analysis for Hospital Management* (Rockville, Maryland: Aspen Publishers, 1984), pp. 291–322.

7.

Teleradiology

Description of the Technology

Teleradiology systems transmit x-ray, CT, MRI, and other images from the imaging centers and radiology/imaging departments where they are created to other places, using telephone lines, microwave transmission, and optical fiber cabling.

The benefits of teleradiology systems include the following:

— The ability to provide an interpretation (or a consultation on an interpretation) without requiring the radiologist to travel to where the image was taken. This can mean a faster response to emergency cases, especially in bad weather.

— The ability to provide the referring physician with access to an image without having to send the film, which would make it unavailable to other physicians who might need it. (No such problem exists, of course, with CT and MRI images that are stored in a computer.)

— The ability to provide the patient who uses a mobile or satellite imaging facility with a fast interpretation without requiring the radiologist to be on-site.

An organization considering the purchase of a system needs to work very carefully with its radiologists and other physicians to assure the acceptability of the purchased system for the proposed uses. Some radiologists will not agree to provide a final interpretation on the basis of a transmitted image, although they may agree to providing an impression, especially in emergency situations.

The controversy concerns the quality of the image transmitted. Some reduction in the quality of radiographic (i.e., x-rays) images still occurs when basic systems are used. Radiologists differ on the importance of this loss in making an interpretation. Those concerned with any loss in image quality may not agree to preparing a final written interpretation until they have seen the film itself.

The transmission of MRI, CT, and images from some nuclear medicine procedures does not automatically result in a reduction in the quality of the image. Theoretically, radiologists and other physicians should not have any objection to providing final interpretations based on images transmitted by basic systems that do not degrade the image. However, the widely known fact that many teleradiology systems do not produce an exact duplicate of a chest x-ray or other radiographic image may result in some reluctance on the part of physicians. Health care organizations need to work with physicians to assure that they will agree to use the equipment required for enough procedures to produce an acceptable level of benefits. It is also important to review with a knowledgeable attorney the legal issues surrounding teleradiology and to explain the issues involved to physicians.

Description of a Basic System

A basic system consists of a sending unit and a receiving unit. Both are usually personal computers, either specially designed units or commercially available equipment. Hard disk drives may or may not be included, depending on the system selected. Both units are equipped with modems to allow the transmission of data over telephone lines. A video camera with the sending unit is attached to a viewing box like the one used by physicians who are reading films.

Enhancements

The enhancements that are available include the following:

— A scan rate converter that allows the transmission of images from CT, MRI, and other devices that produce a high resolution (i.e., extremely detailed) image in a computer, but not on film. Without a converter, such images must be placed on film and then scanned by the video camera with some loss in sharpness. This process also requires additional training of technicians in framing, focusing, and cropping the film image.

— A variety of display monitors that vary in resolution and ability to receive color signals. Some workstations may have multiple screens to allow the viewing of multiple images at the same time.

— Optical laser disk storage that allows for the storage of many images. Computers linked to this storage unit can search for and retrieve any image desired.

— Voice and/or text transmission with an image. The system may automatically "toggle" (i.e., move back and forth between) text and image, or provide "on-screen annotation" (i.e., the text appears on the image). Voice transmission can be with the image or separately.

— Transmission over optical fiber networks, by microwave, or both. Optical fiber cables allow for faster transmission of images than over telephone lines, and with no loss of data. The sending and receiving stations must be linked, however, by this type of cable. It is now most frequently used to link two points in a building or several buildings (for example, on the campus of a medical center). Microwave transmission also permits (with no loss of data) faster image transmission than over telephone lines. However, the two points to be linked must have an unobstructed view of each other since transmissions cannot be made through buildings and other obstacles. Satellite transmission is now becoming available as an alternative (see Exhibit 7.5).

The "Purchase or Develop" Decision

The specialized software required for teleradiology systems is not available from retail computer stores, and most staff and consultants who are familiar with personal computer software will have no experience with the special requirements of this type of programming. For almost all health care organizations, developing a system internally is not a realistic alternative.

Expertise on how to make the various pieces of hardware work well with each other is also likely to be missing. This will make it difficult for health care organizations to purchase hardware such as personal computers from its normal suppliers and try to link them with the video cameras and scan rate converters used in these systems. Vendors sell these systems as packages and service them as systems.

Potential for Enhancing Services

Teleradiology systems can transmit x-ray, MRI, and CT images to a physician over telephone lines for interpretation, reducing some of the travel required to provide this service to a hospital or physician group practice on nights and weekends. Since radiologists can provide an interpretation in their homes or offices, speed and accuracy are improved. The purchase and use of this technology could also improve patient perceptions of the conscientiousness or professionalism of physicians. It can also improve access to the service in areas where radiologists are not available.

Teleradiology can also be used to provide physicians and patients access to the expertise of specialists regardless of where they are located, without always requiring the patient to travel. Patients may no longer need to travel to a regional center for some procedures.

The practices of referring physicians are also supported. Physicians with access to receiving equipment can easily receive images taken elsewhere and can have images produced locally (for example, in a group practice's own imaging center) interpreted by a specialist at a remote site.

The ways in which teleradiology might provide an imaging center or hospital imaging/radiology department with a competitive advantage have been discussed in more detail by Alexander Szafran and Roger Kropf.[1]

Examples

Multiple Uses and Benefits

Exhibit 7.1 is a description of a basic teleradiology system which sold in 1989 for under $25,000. Exhibits 7.2 and 7.3 describe some of the uses of this system:

— To save radiologists time and to avoid having them travel in unsafe conditions

— To increase the speed with which an interpretation can be provided, especially in emergency situations and when a mobile imaging unit is involved

— To allow for consultations at any time with any specialist with access to the technology

Exhibit 7.4 suggests that teleradiology may also have some indirect benefits. By providing access to specialized expertise, a rural health care organization may help in the recruitment and retention of all types of physicians, but especially those who would not consider rural practice because they do not believe good medicine can be practiced without the help of physicians in other specialties.

Exhibit 7.5 illustrates how combining teleradiology with other technologies may provide even greater benefits. For example, a voice recognition system customized for radiologists is being used to turn a dictated interpretation directly into printed text. Using mobile imaging equipment and satellite transmission, services can now be provided without the patient traveling, but with a quick turnaround of the report.

Exhibit 7.1   Advertisement for the Photophone® Teleradiology System

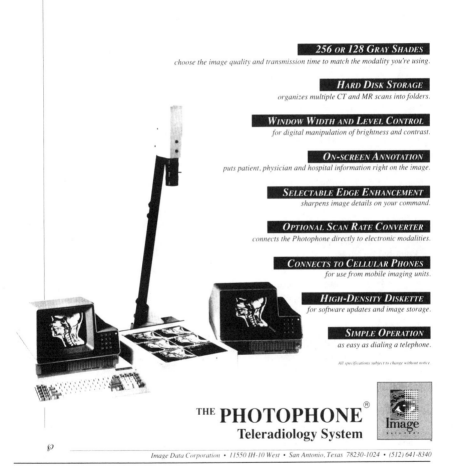

INTRODUCING
Affordable, Full-featured Teleradiology That's Easy to Use

256 OR 128 GRAY SHADES
choose the image quality and transmission time to match the modality you're using.

HARD DISK STORAGE
organizes multiple CT and MR scans into folders.

WINDOW WIDTH AND LEVEL CONTROL
for digital manipulation of brightness and contrast.

ON-SCREEN ANNOTATION
puts patient, physician and hospital information right on the image.

SELECTABLE EDGE ENHANCEMENT
sharpens image details on your command.

OPTIONAL SCAN RATE CONVERTER
connects the Photophone directly to electronic modalities.

CONNECTS TO CELLULAR PHONES
for use from mobile imaging units.

HIGH-DENSITY DISKETTE
for software updates and image storage.

SIMPLE OPERATION
as easy as dialing a telephone.

All specifications subject to change without notice.

THE **PHOTOPHONE**®
Teleradiology System   Image

Image Data Corporation • 11550 IH-10 West • San Antonio, Texas 78230-1024 • (512) 641-8340

Source: Reprinted with the permission of Image Data Corporation, San Antonio, Texas.

Exhibit 7.2   Advertisement for Photophone®

THE   PHOTOPHONE   AT   WORK
Richmond Memorial Hospital:
Beating The Clock For Better Patient Care

Hospital:	*Service Provided:*
Richmond Memorial Hospital	**Diagnosis of medical images**
Location:	*Photophone Application:*
Staten Island, New York	**Teleradiology**

The legendary race against time. We're all faced with it and, as always, man is consumed with beating it. Particularly in the medical arena where saving lives is fundamentally related to saving time.

Thanks to new technology called teleradiology, doctors at Richmond Memorial Hospital, a division of Community Health System of Staten Island, have found a way to beat the clock and improve the delivery of their radiological services at the same time.

Fact is, this small community hospital is just one of many nationwide now using the Photophone MD-1 teleradiology system developed by Image Data Corporation of San Antonio. The Photophone improves response times by transmitting medical images over normal phone lines.

Now when patients are brought into the hospital in the middle of the night, radiologists are able to respond almost instantly—from miles away! And in a congested urban area like New York City, response like that is virtually unheard of.

"In an emergency situation, city traffic or weather can increase our response time beyond acceptable limits," says Dr. Sapienza who purchased the MD-1 system with colleague Dr. Daniel Carfora. "Waiting for one of us to make the 45-minute commute is the last thing a critically injured patient needs. Sometimes, a few minutes saved in trauma cases can mean the difference between living and dying."

But teleradiology has changed that picture. Now when the phone rings at 4 a.m., the icy bridge separating Sapienza's Brooklyn home and Staten Island's Richmond Memorial hospital no longer interferes with getting his job done. Technologists at the hospital simply send medical images over phone lines directly to the Photophone MD-1 unit at Sapienza's home. Ordinarily, transmission takes just about 15 to 20 seconds.

Richmond Memorial has augmented the MD-1 system with an optional video interface which converts images generated by their CT scanner (CAT scans) to a video signal the Photophone can recognize.

"It's worked flawlessly," says Dr. Sapienza, "and we don't have to convert images from a digital format to film and back."

Dr. Sapienza says there's little doubt that teleradiology is quickly becoming the most cost-effective way to bring the doctor to the studies—at a moment's notice—without the hassles of trying to beat the clock!

"The MD-1 has really performed, and diagnostically, we're very comfortable with its resolution," says Dr. Sapienza. "When you compare its image quality and low cost with other products currently on the market, it works well for us."

Finally, the race against time is over—at least for the patients of radiologists who use teleradiology.

Continued

Exhibit 7.2   Continued

The Problem	Photophone Solution
Before teleradiology,	*With teleradiology,*
• *there was no substitute for the radiologist's presence at the hospital to study images*	• *the number of nighttime trips to the hospital are reduced*
• *the radiologists spent many hours driving to and from hospitals, often at late hours*	• *decisions are made quickly*
	• *radiologists can consult simultaneously on multiple cases at multiple hospitals*

Source: Reprinted with the permission of Image Data Corporation, San Antonio, Texas.

The Financial Payoff

Teleradiology systems themselves do not generate additional revenue. The major financial questions are whether they result in greater use of the service by patients and referring physicians, a competitive advantage in negotiations with third-party payers and self-insured employers, and an increase in the satisfaction of radiologists and staff physicians that lowers costs (for example, by lowering staff turnover and, therefore, recruitment costs).

No studies of such a financial impact were uncovered in the research for this chapter. Vendors are primarily concerned about physician satisfaction, rather than demonstrating financial impact. This may be a reflection of their belief that managers and boards of health care organizations will make a purchase because it is likely to lead to greater physician satisfaction. It may also be because the cost of a basic teleradiology system is relatively low. It would also be difficult to attribute a decision by patients and physicians to use a health care facility to an improvement in one ancillary service.

Selecting the Components of a System

A basic system is sold as a unit. As mentioned earlier, it is unlikely that most health care organizations will have staff with the expertise to assemble the hardware for a system or do the necessary programming.

A major question for many health care organizations considering monitors, optical disk storage, and other enhancements will be whether to

Exhibit 7.3   Description of Photophone® Application

Photophone® Application

Ten Radiologists Agree on Diagnosis: Photophone Helps

It might be difficult to get a group of radiologists to agree on patient care or the most effective treatment procedure. But, after a three-month evaluation at Lutheran General Hospital, all 10 staff radiologists agree that the Photophone video telephone is a big help in their work.

The Photophone video telephone sends images, such as X-rays, over a standard phone line in seconds.

"We use the Photophone as an on-call unit," says Jean-Claude Harris, radiological engineer at the Park Ridge, Ill. hospital. "Whoever is on call takes the Photophone home with him. Then, if we have a trauma case in the middle of the night, we can send the X-rays directly to the radiologist's house. It usually saves him a trip to the hospital."

It took three months for the 800-bed hospital to evaluate the Photophone because Harris wanted each radiologist to get a chance to use it during the week he was on call.

The Photophone won accolades for its seven-second transmission; its ability to store 20 images in internal memory; its portability; and its ease of use. The standard Photophone is already equipped with features designed specifically for radiologists; it can zoom in on a picture, step up an image's contrast and produce "negative" video images.

Lutheran General has two Photophones now and plans to use more in the future, Harris said.

"We have 64 acres of hospital grounds here with several satellite clinics at various locations," he said. "It's difficult for our radiology department to do it all."

With Photophones, the satellite clinics could send X-rays to the main radiology department for viewing. The department could also use the video telephones to send an image of an X-ray back to the clinic so the patient's own physician could view them.

Another potential use for the Photophones at Lutheran General is for specialized radiology.

"Radiology is becoming a field of specialization. You'll have neuro-radiologists and pediatric radiologists," Harris said. "If you give each of the specialists a Photophone for permanent use, they could easily be consulted, if an injury demands a specialist's attention."

While attending the 1986 North American Radiology Show, Harris checked other tele-radiology equipment. (Tele-radiology involves transmitting X-rays over the telephone lines to a remote site.)

"For its price, its features and its ease of use, the Photophone couldn't be beat," he said.

Image Data Corp. created the first practical video telephone more than two years ago and has sold hundreds of Photophones to the nation's top corporations. Headed by managers with more than 50 years of corporate marketing and engineering experience, the San Antonio company maintains a nationwide sales and support network.

Source: Reprinted with the permission of Image Data Corporation, San Antonio, Texas.

Exhibit 7.4 Teleradiology May Ease Rural Staffing Problems

It hasn't been easy for hospitals in western Nebraska to recruit physicians. Few people are attracted to small-town life in an isolated region. And when it comes to physician recruitment, hardscrabble economics and a sparse population aren't the only deterrents.

"Most doctors are trained in an urban setting with a lot of subspecialty backup," says Shauna Libsack, director of physician relations for West Nebraska General Hospital, a 228-bed facility in Scottsbluff. "There's a certain amount of insecurity that comes with isolation from your colleagues."

Nebraska isn't the only place where there are recruitment problems. More than 1,900 communities across the country are in dire need of primary medical care. To make matters worse, it is feared that regulation of physician fees will make it more difficult to lure doctors to rural areas, according to Robert Van Hook, executive director of the National Rural Health Association, Kansas City, MO.

Technology helps. But staffing problems in rural radiology departments may be eased with the help of teleradiology, a technology that can transmit radiographic images from one computer to another within moments. With teleradiology, radiologists in a distant location can make a primary diagnosis from an image or consult with a specialist about the findings.

Using a newly purchased teleradiology system, West Nebraska General is providing consultation services to smaller hospitals in the region. West Nebraska General hopes that the program will generate more patient referrals from neighboring hospitals, Libsack explains. Smaller hospitals that link into the teleradiology system gain subspecialty support that could help them recruit physicians, Libsack adds.

Teleradiology linkages could help hospitals of any size that lack medical staff in certain specialties. "In nuclear medicine, full-time practitioners don't exist at the community level. Hospitals that want to offer the service often don't have access to the expertise they need," says Robert Henkin, M.D., director of nuclear medicine at Loyola University Medical Center, Maywood, IL.

Henkin helped develop a teleradiology package called Nuclear Image Transmission Software (NITS) that transmits nuclear medicine images across telephone lines to any NITS user with a personal computer. In addition, six physicians at major teaching facilities are available through the network to interpret images and do consultation.

Sticky points. Some radiologists question the quality of images transmitted through teleradiology. At West Nebraska General, for example, "Our radiologists will do a preliminary assessment of an image, but they insist on seeing the original film before they make a final decision," Libsack says.

But "teleradiology can provide images of primary diagnostic quality," says Jay Wheeler, M.D., associate dean for medical education and special programs at Texas Tech Health Sciences Center, Lubbock. For example, Vortech Data, Inc., Richardson, TX, provides high-speed transmission of finely detailed images by satellite to the Hospital of the University of Pennsylvania, Pittsburgh, where primary diagnoses are made from the images.

Wheeler is currently at work on a federally funded study of the impact telecommunications could have on health care in underserved regions.

Laura Souhrada

Exhibit 7.5 Radiology via Phone and Satellite

Patients in remote locations can now be studied by radiologists, thanks to a combination of state-of-the-art communications technology, Kurzweil VoiceRAD systems—and vans.

Some health care authorities believe this procedure—called "teleradiology"—will be an increasingly common way to perform radiological studies; it is generally faster, safer, more convenient and cheaper than bringing the patient into a radiology department.

Two different firms in the Los Angeles area now dispatch vans filled with X-ray equipment to rest homes, rehabilitation and convalescent centers, clinics and private homes. Medical technicians then take X-ray films of a patient, and transmit them electronically—by satellite or over phone lines—to a radiologist many miles away at teleradiology headquarters.

The radiologist then studies the transmitted X-ray, dictates a report into a Kurzweil VoiceRAD system, and transmits it—either by the same satellite route or an ordinary phone line—back to the mobile unit. There, the report is printed out for a referring physician or health care worker, who can then administer appropriate care to the patient.

The satellite system is run by Professional Satellite Imaging, located in Colton, California. The other company—which depends on phone lines and modems for transmitting information—is called Remote Imaging System and is located in Anaheim, California.

Dan L. Wilbanks, vice president of Remote Imaging Systems, began setting up his firm's teleradiology business seven years ago—prior to the availability of Kurzweil AI's technology.

"But we always planned on incorporating voice into the system," he says. "Voice recognition is a real step forward. In teleradiology, as in other forms of radiology, voice recognition gets fast, accurate information from the radiologist to the referring physician."

Source: Kurzweil Applied Intelligence, Inc., "Radiology via Phone and Satellite," *VoiceMED* (Winter 1988–89), p. 3. Reprinted with the permission of Kurzweil AI, Waltham, Massachusetts.

move toward the development of a Picture Archiving and Communications Systems (PACS), or to assure that the teleradiology system purchased is compatible with one.

PACS systems combine rapid image transmission (especially image transmission within a facility), computer storage of most images, software and hardware for rapid retrieval and manipulation of images, and a network of computers and monitors to allow access to the images. To achieve the desired speed, optical fiber cabling (which transmit signals as light) and optical laser disk storage (which use laser beams to store data on disks, much like a commercial compact audio disk) are often considered essential.

Although a basic teleradiology system can be purchased for under $25,000, a PACS system could easily cost a hospital more than a million dollars. Both teleradiology and PACS systems are designed to transmit images, but with vastly different objectives. The objectives of PACS systems are to achieve the benefits of storing and transmitting most images in digital form (zeros and ones), rather than as film. Basic teleradiology systems are not intended to provide libraries of images for later use by physicians, but access to selected images that are needed at a particular moment.

The subject of PACS is important because managers who are considering the use of teleradiology will have to consider whether a PACS system will be implemented in the near future. The vendors of PACS systems also offer teleradiology as part of their PACS system, but their equipment is likely to be incompatible with the basic systems on the market.

Given the low cost of basic systems, the issue of compatibility should not affect the decision to purchase a few basic systems. However, organizations that are considering tying together a network of clinics, hospitals, physicians' offices, and other facilities need to consider if it will be possible to integrate a teleradiology system into a PACS system at a later date.

Note

1. Alexander J. Szafran and Roger Kropf, "Strategic Uses of Teleradiology," *Radiology Management* 10, no. 2 (Spring 1988) : 23–27.

Part III

Deciding Which Technologies
to Invest In

8.

Criteria for Selecting Computer Technologies

The major questions facing health care managers considering the acquisition of these technologies are:

1. Do they provide the specific results that vendors claim?
2. Do the results justify the costs involved?
3. Can combinations of these technologies greatly improve the results?

The validation of each vendor's claims must be made by the individual purchaser through a process of investigation that includes actually viewing the system in operation in similar health care organizations. Developing criteria for making a selection is an important step to assure that any review of the technology does not focus just on what a vendor believes are the technology's strengths. Criteria that could be used to assess the value of a technology are presented in this chapter to help in the development of an organization's own criteria for selection, which must be based on the organization's own goals and capabilities.

Table 8.1 lists some of the criteria that could be used to make a decision on whether to purchase an individual technology. In Chapter 9, these criteria are applied to a specific technology to illustrate how the criteria might be used.

Who Benefits?

1. Who will primarily benefit?   Most technologies offer benefits for several groups. For example, a computer link that allows for remote scheduling of a

Table 8.1   Acquiring Technology for Service Enhancement: Questions
for Managers

Who Benefits?

1. Who will primarily benefit? Patients? Referring physicians? Referral physicians?

Will Utilization Be Affected?

2. What role do they play in determining if your services are used? Primary or secondary decision makers?

3. What are the expected benefits? How large will they be? Time and/or money saved? Increase in perceived service quality? Is a new, valued service created?

4. Are benefits of this magnitude known to be important in the decision to use your services? Known to be extremely important, secondary, marginal? Confirmed by research, suspected, unknown?

5. Could providing the benefits differentiate you from competitors or reduce their competitive advantage?

Is the Proposed Use Ethical and Legal?

6. Will the proposed program be viewed as unethical?

7. Is the proposed program legal?

Can You Sustain the Competitive Advantage?

8. How easy will it be for competitors to implement the technology and reduce any competitive advantage? Is the technology itself easy to acquire? Are the other resources used easy to obtain, such as staff and medical specialists? Will the use of the technology raise substantial barriers to entry for potential competitors?

9. Is being first to use the technology and offer its benefits likely to lead to consumer loyalty, high switching costs for consumers, or both?

Continued

procedure benefits patients, referring physicians and their office staff, and the organization providing the service. Each group does not benefit equally, however, and determining the perceived importance of the actual benefits provided will move the organization closer to determining whether the technology should be purchased. Patients who have never tried to schedule the procedure before may perceive little added value to the computer link, for example, although office staff treasure the new ease and speed.

Will Utilization Be Affected?

2. What role do they play in determining if your services are used?   If the group or individual that makes the decision on the use of services perceives the technology to add significant value to a service, the technology may result in higher utilization. If the group has little influence over the choice, it may not.

For example, if pregnant women perceive remote scheduling to add

Table 8.1 Continued

Evaluation

10. What is the relationship between cost and expected benefits? Is expected new volume × net revenue per unit > cost? Cost justifiable to reduce anxiety about market share decline?

11. Can you (or the vendor) put in place a system for continuous monitoring of changes in service volume? Does it question customers about the importance of the benefits provided?

12. Will a system be put in place that monitors the behavioral impact of the technology on staff, patients, and physicians? Does increasing the flow of information change behavior? Does substituting a computer link for a face-to-face encounter alter job or service satisfaction?

Implementation

13. Is anyone in your organization responsible and accountable for service quality? Do they have the authority to institute change?

14. Do the responsible parties have the knowledge, willingness, and skills to acquire and install the technology? If they lack skills and knowledge will someone, inside or outside of the organization, support them?

15. Will your organization commit the resources to train and motivate front-line people (for example, nurses) to use and support the technology?

16. Is the use of technology part of a larger effort to make service quality a superordinate goal of the organization? Are there motivated front-line people trying to alter their behavior whom the technology can support? Is management making a personal commitment to change?

---

little to a service (for example, labor and delivery), it is unlikely to affect the choice of hospital. Some women follow their physician's advice; others have a strongly held set of values about how this service should be provided. The obstetrician's office staff, however, may feel that remote scheduling has made a significant improvement in their work lives. Although the value added is real and significant to the office staff, significant numbers of women could use their own networks of peers to seek out information and select a hospital that is willing to meet their perceived needs.

3. What are the expected benefits? How large will they be?   The benefits offered by the technology are of different types (see Tables 1.1 and 1.2) and magnitudes. Time may be saved, allowing patients to pursue other leisure or work activities. Money may be saved for the health care organization because salaries do not have to be paid for workers as volume increases. The benefits may be psychological; for example, physicians' perceptions of their worth to the organization may be enhanced by receiving access to information through a computer link.

Although the benefits may be perceived as real, they may also be perceived as being large or insignificantly small. A physician who receives a computer to use in scheduling hospital services may perceive a real benefit to staff but feel that because it does not allow the office to run with fewer staff (one secretary/receptionist being needed at all times), the benefits are not significant.

The benefits may increase the perceived quality of an existing service or help create a new service package. Second opinions via a teleradiology network create a new service not previously available; a teleradiology network that permits a radiologist to read images at a hospital without driving there provides significant benefits for the radiologist offering an existing service.

The benefits must not only be identified, but also measured. They can be measured through surveys on perceived benefits, by observing behavior before and after the implementation of the technology, or by experiments that involve providing the technology to a group of physicians or patients and observing the differences in behavior when compared to a group that did not have access.

4. Are benefits of this magnitude **known** *to be important in the decision to use your services?*   The benefits provided may be known to be extremely important, secondary, or of marginal importance. Some "knowledge," however, is merely conjecture sanctified by constant repetition in conversations and in publications.

Many radiology departments and imaging centers have adopted a policy, for example, of transmitting films (or digital images through teleradiology) to referring physicians along with an interpretation within 24 hours of the image/film being taken. The assumption is that referring physicians value the speed. Other departments/centers telephone positive reports, but transmit negative ones through the regular mails, assuming that physicians are unlikely to see their patients within a day of a film/image being taken, especially for a routine exam such as a chest x-ray or mammogram. Who's right? It is hard to deny that physicians who order a service like speed, and they may perceive that a service has been enhanced. This does not mean that they will change their behavior or remain loyal to a particular provider. Other considerations, including their investment in a particular organization and personal relationships with other physicians, could have a greater effect on which service they use. Factors influencing physician and patient decision making need to be examined through observation of behavior, focus groups, and interviews.

5. Could providing the benefits differentiate you from competitors or reduce their competitive advantage?   Some components of a service package are needed to meet, rather than exceed, the value of services offered by competitors. Other enhancements serve to differentiate a service from what is offered by competitors. Meeting the competition may be extremely important to prevent a loss of market share but will not increase the volume of services used. It is important to understand this distinction in order to reduce the disappointment that may arise when the enhancement of services fails to increase volume.

A technology that allows an organization to meet and exceed the value offered by a competitor's service is, therefore, extremely valuable. A computer link that meets a competitor's standard for report turnaround and offers second opinions from respected specialists presents the possibility of growth, as opposed to just maintenance, of market share.

Is the Proposed Use Ethical and Legal?

6. Will the proposed program be viewed as unethical?   Some benefits are real and measurable and will affect the use of services, but obtaining them may violate values held by groups in the organization or may violate the law. Some of those values can be described by the following statements:

— No physician or other provider of services should personally profit from a referral for a service, since the patient's welfare should be the primary goal in making such decisions.

— A health care organization's role is to provide treatment when requested, rather than to stimulate demand for its services through active outreach solely for the purpose of achieving higher revenues.

These are not the only values that some individuals or groups may feel will be violated. Managers will need to raise the issue of ethics and values in discussing each proposed program to assure that implementation of any program that is eventually developed is not jeopardized by active or passive resistance as a result of feelings that the program is unethical.

For example, when a group of physicians feels that the hospital's standing in the community as an organization with the highest ethical values is being violated by an active outbound telemarketing campaign, it can result in efforts to reduce or eliminate the budget for the program (active resistance) and quiet discussion among physicians of the low quality of the services being offered (more passive resistance), regardless of whether the quality of the program is known.

Another major area of concern is the provision of free goods or services to physicians with the objective of increasing their referrals for services. A hospital could provide physicians with free fax machines, with the expectation that lab and other orders would increase because results would be returned faster. Since the machines cost money and can be used by the physician for their own purposes, they may be viewed as an additional payment for referrals. This is likely to offend some managers, clinicians, and members of the board of trustees who believe that physicians should not profit from the referral of patients because it alters the role of the physician as an advocate for the patient's welfare.

Although consensus on values cannot always be achieved, who objects, and why, needs to be understood by managers in order to allow the communication of information to dispel rumors and misunderstanding, and to organize discussion of the program to determine if changes could be made that could reduce the objections. Outbound telemarketing could be limited to potential patients who indicated on a survey form or response card that they were interested in receiving information on a service. The fax machines could be sold to physicians by a local retailer who agreed to give each physician the same discount it would offer to the hospital for a large-volume purchase. The fax machines could also be leased to the physicians for a low monthly rate, with no requirement that they be purchased at the end of the lease. The low cost and other uses to which the machine could be put might make the offer very attractive to physicians.

7. Is the proposed program legal?   Providing free or subsidized hardware, software, or services to physicians or other providers who refer Medicare or Medicaid patients may also be in violation of the fraud and abuse regulations of the federal government and some state governments, which bar the exchange of anything of value in return for the referral of a patient.[1] What constitutes fraud and abuse is now being debated in the Congress, the federal bureaucracy, and the courts. There are currently no "safe harbors" (i.e., programs that are automatically legal) that involve providing physicians with goods or services. Any program needs to be reviewed by legal counsel. This is not meant to suggest that providing any goods or services to physicians at less-than-retail prices is automatically unethical or illegal. If the amount of the benefit offered is not related to the volume of patients referred, it may still be legal. A hospital that provides a fax machine through a subsidized lease to *all* physicians on the medical staff who request one may not be in violation of federal and state fraud and abuse laws.

Another legal issue is "inurement," that is, the use of the resources of a not-for-profit organization for private gain. Again, legal counsel is essential in determining whether the provision of goods and services violates state law or federal tax codes. If the tax-exempt purposes of the organization (the delivery of health services) are served by the program, and physicians make fair payments for the use of the tax-exempt organization's resources, there may be no problem.[2] In addition to legal problems, stories in the newspaper or on television that suggest that a not-for-profit organization is using its resources for the private gain of physicians and other providers could have negative consequences for the organization's fund-raising campaigns and its requests before various regulatory bodies.

Health care organizations that undertake active outbound telemarketing also need to become aware of the local and state regulations concerning telephone and personal solicitation. The rights of the consumer and the responsibilities of the vendor need to be understood, and any necessary changes made in the program being marketed.

These are only a few examples of the importance of obtaining legal counsel. Others include the need to explore the regulations governing microwave transmission (to establish telecommunications links) and the need to consider laws and regulations concerning the confidentiality of patient medical records before they are used for purposes other than medical care (for example, outbound telemarketing).

Can You Sustain the Competitive Advantage?

8. How easy will it be for competitors to implement the technology and reduce any competitive advantage? If the technology itself is easy to acquire, a competitor could negate any competitive advantage by using it to enhance its service package. Cost is one measure of ease of acquisition, with cost broadly defined to include the purchase price and the cost of implementation and operation. It is important to examine implementation costs carefully since the recruitment and training of staff, data base development, and systems testing involved in computer technologies can easily cost far more than the original acquisition price.

The resources required to use the technology, such as staff and physical facilities, may not be easy to obtain. A referral service that offers access to registered nurses over the telephone may be difficult to implement in an area with a severe nursing shortage, for example. Respected specialists who could provide second opinions after reviewing test reports and images transmitted by satellite or over the telephone may not be available locally.

The cost of using technology to enhance a service and the scarcity of the necessary resources can both raise significant barriers to entry for potential competitors. To enter the market, in this case by offering the enhanced service that patients and physicians now expect, these barriers must be overcome. For some potential competitors, the barriers will appear so high that they will choose not to offer the service, reducing competition that could lower profitability. A competitive advantage is built on both the loyalty of physicians and patients and the unwillingness of competitors to meet or exceed the service package being offered and win market share. An organization considering the acquisition of technology to win a competitive advantage should consider whether the resulting barriers to entry will be high.

9. Is being first to use the technology and offer its benefits likely to lead to consumer loyalty, high switching costs for consumers, or both?   Offering a new or enhanced service *first* is sometimes done with the expectation that a competitive advantage will automatically result. Some barriers to entry are created by being first, but as Michael Porter[3] has noted, there are some disadvantages to early entry into a market. Acquisition of scarce resources is one possible barrier to entry that is created. A multiyear, exclusive consulting agreement between an organization and a noted medical specialist to provide consultations is one example. However, such agreements are expensive and difficult to negotiate.

Another barrier to entry is both patient and physician loyalty and/or "switching costs" that they incur by changing to another service. Loyalty is, of course, voluntary, and both patients and physicians will feel obligated to switch to a health care organization that they perceive to offer high-quality services. Some costs are incurred, however, in switching. The enhancement of a service by a competitor may be counterbalanced by the continual innovations of an organization that understands patient and physician needs better because of its longer experience.

For example, a freestanding cancer treatment center that is the first to offer services may quickly find that it faces competition. Because it was first to serve its market, however, it may have developed in a computer data base a profile of the practices of the physicians it serves, including the present problems of their patients. It could use this information to customize its mail to these physicians, offering them case studies of the effective diagnosis and treatment of problems that they frequently face.

The new competitor lacks this information. The physician who considers changing to a competing center will suffer a switching cost, that is, the cost of not having this information to aid in clinical practice. Some physicians will consider this cost insignificant, but if other costs are involved, the result can be a loyalty built on self-interest.

Organizations considering the acquisition of technology need to consider if the switching costs that will result will be high or low. The higher they are, the more likely the organization will develop a sustainable competitive advantage.

Evaluation

10. What is the relationship between cost and expected benefits?   This is probably the major question asked by managers, but as the previous discussion suggests, the answer can be difficult to discover. One formula for determining this relationship would be

$$\text{expected new volume} \times \text{net revenue per unit} > \text{cost}$$

Historical data can suggest some possible results. If each additional referral of a patient yields $100 in net revenue, then an investment whose annualized cost is $200,000 requires an increase of 2,000 patients per year to reach breakeven; an investment of $20,000, an increase of 200 patients. Examination of the size of the total existing demand, a projection of unserved demand, and assumptions about reasonable short-term shifts in market share will suggest the magnitude of investment that should be considered. The same logic might be applied to losses in market share. How many referrals would we have to lose to justify the investment?

The calculations are even more complicated because the technology may attract new patients and physicians with different costs and net revenues. It may also create a new service for which the potential demand is unknown. The enhancement of the service may also create a barrier to entry that keeps out a potential competitor whose entry into the market might have devastating effects, rather than resulting in a small loss of market share.

The immediate reaction may be to invest small and slowly, but as the preceding discussion suggests, small enhancements are likely to raise few barriers to entry and create low switching costs.

The amount of market research conducted should reflect the size of the investment being considered and provide a firm base for making these decisions. For a large investment, surveys and other research should be carried out to find out how patients and physicians perceive the organization's service, and its competitors', what enhancements they might value, and the factors they consider in making a purchase decision, among other topics.

11. Can you (or the vendor) put in place a system for continuous monitoring of changes in service volume? Does it question customers about the importance of the benefits provided? Acquisition and implementation of the technology should be just the beginning of research. While some research will continue to be through surveys and other original data collection, the technology itself can generate much useful information. For example, a computer system for scheduling services and reporting results can yield information on who orders what services and when. The collection and analysis of such data to produce useful information should be part of the service package offered by the vendor of the technology, or should be developed by the organization as a last resort.

12. Will a system be put in place that monitors the behavioral impact of the technology on staff, patients, and physicians? The installation of a computer system can have major consequences for how people in health care organizations behave, and some of the changes are not positive, as Mari Malvey[4] and Shoshana Zuboff[5] describe in great detail.

No formal research has been done on the impact of using the technologies described in this book in health care organizations. The assumption should not be made that all impacts will be positive.

For example, increasing the flow of information within and between organizations could change behavior. A lab technician, aware that a computer-based system is monitoring the flow of work to reduce patient and physician waiting time, may cooperate and suggest improvements in work flow, or actively obstruct the system in a variety of ways. Obstructions could include deliberately entering incorrect data to show the system does not work, continually criticizing the system to encourage coworkers not to use it, and maintaining manual systems purporting to show the computer system is wrong.

Substituting a computer link for a face-to-face encounter could alter job or service satisfaction. The telephone call or face-to-face encounter that used to occur to transfer information or to make a request served a number of other functions, some very positive for both the organization and the individual. One of these is to transfer unrelated, but important, information about the functioning of the organization and its members. For example, information could be transmitted on the status of labor negotiations, requests for purchases of new equipment, and other subjects of vital interest to staff.

How can these effects be discovered? Although formal research—surveys and systematic interviews—are sometimes necessary, it is also important that the organization continually monitor the effects of new technology. This could include the selection of performance measures that might serve as indicators of acceptance of the new technology: error rates in data entry are an example. Building questions on the use of technology into performance reviews and other personnel actions is another example. Inviting an outside observer to visit the organization and look at how the technology is being used could provide a useful external viewpoint. In this way, management can develop a plan for implementation that prevents and reduces negative consequences, while helping to assure that the organization realizes the benefits it expected.

Implementation

13. Is anyone in your organization responsible and accountable for service quality? Do they have the authority to institute change? Karl Albrecht and Ron Zemke[6] emphasize that service quality has to be managed. When no one is in charge—responsible and accountable—the result is a decline into mediocrity. Support must come from the very top of the organization, although a group could be empowered to develop and implement the necessary plans to raise the level of quality. This group must have the authority, however, to assure that the plans developed and approved are carried out.

This is easy to say and difficult to carry out, since service excellence requires the active participation of many people in the organization. Karl Albrecht[7] and Jan Carlzon[8] have offered many suggestions on how to develop an organizational structure. In the end, someone—a group or individual—needs to be responsible and accountable and have the active support and participation of the head of the organization.

14. Do the responsible parties have the knowledge, willingness, and skills to acquire and install the technology?   If the individual or group responsible for improving service quality lacks the skills and knowledge to design and implement changes, someone—inside or outside of the organization—will be needed to support them by providing training and advice. A number of consulting firms have made this a specialty and should be considered at appropriate points to avoid duplicating the effort involved in certain activities, for example, designing training programs, and to avoid mistakes made in other organizations. It should be emphasized, however, that the effort to improve service quality cannot be turned over to an outside consultant. As Albrecht[9] notes, significant improvement in service quality will take several years in most organizations, and consultant involvement for more than short periods is extremely expensive and ineffective if no one in the organization has committed themselves to the effort by devoting significant amounts of time to it.

The use of technology may, of course, require the use of specialists in computers and telecommunications from outside of the organization. Any contract that is signed to acquire a technology should carefully stipulate the level of effort to be made by the vendor to make the system operational, state penalties for failure to meet performance standards in a specific time period, and describe the services (and the cost of those services) available for modifying the system at the later date to meet organizational needs and take advantage of software and hardware advances.

15. Will your organization commit the resources to train and motivate front-line people (for example, nurses) to use and support the technology? Training and support costs are frequently underestimated by organizations that acquire computer technology. The tendency is to focus on the purchase price, rather than the total costs of acquisition and implementation. An estimate should be made prior to acquisition of the training cost involved, including an estimate of the need for additional training based on staff turnover, which can be high in health care organizations. If those costs seem too high, a more limited implementation of the technology should be undertaken. Failure to train and motivate those who will operate the technology is a major reason why organizations fail to realize the benefits they expected.

For example, failure to adequately train office staff to use a computer link to schedule hospital services will result in some patients being given a telephone number and asked to make the appointment themselves, negating the benefit of enhanced patient satisfaction that was expected.

16. Is the use of technology part of a larger effort to make service quality a superordinate goal of the organization?   Tom Peters and Robert Waterman, Jr., stressed the importance of "superordinate goals" in explaining why some organizations succeed in achieving excellence.[10] Carlzon[11] and Albrecht[12] also emphasize that an organization needs one or more goals that can be briefly stated to employees that describe what the organization is trying to achieve.

Technology can serve only to enhance an effort to make service excellence a superordinate goal of the organization. If no such goal exists, then the technology is more likely to be used by unmotivated front-line people who perceive that the organization's purpose is to serve them, their bosses, or the stockholders. Excellent service to patients and physicians is unlikely to result.

There must be motivated front-line people trying to alter their behavior whom the technology can support. As Albrecht[13] notes, a basic change has to occur. Everyone and everything (including computer and telecommunications technology) must directly serve the customer, or someone who does.

A superordinate goal is unlikely to be accepted and influence behavior unless management makes a personal commitment to change. Telling nurses that service to patients and physicians is a superordinate goal of the organization is unlikely to change behavior if they see that management spends most of its time negotiating lower supply prices, examining staff productivity in order to reduce staffing, and worrying about new freestanding services. Although these activities are important, they are unlikely to be viewed as immediately supporting nurses in the job they have been asked to do.

Should All the Criteria Be Used?

The criteria that have just been described will take time and effort to use. How much time management spends should depend on the magnitude of the investment being considered. Large investments should be preceded by more careful consideration of more of the criteria because the risks are higher.

Notes

1. Ann James, "Legal Issues in Physician Bonding," in Stephen Valentine, ed., *Physician Bonding: Developing a Successful Hospital Program* (Rockville, Maryland: Aspen Publishers, 1989), p. 95.

2. Barbara Turner and Leslie Granow, "Joint Ventures as a Bonding Tool" in Stephen Valentine, ed., *Physician Bonding*, p. 123.

3. Michael E. Porter, *Competitive Advantage: Creating and Sustaining Superior Performance* (New York: Free Press, 1985).

4. Mari Malvey, *Simple Systems, Complex Environment: Hospital Financial Information Systems* (Beverly Hills, California: Sage Publications, 1981).

5. Shoshana Zuboff, *In the Age of the Smart Machine: The Future of Work and Power* (New York: Basic Books, 1988).

6. Karl Albrecht and Ron Zemke, *Service America! Doing Business in the New Economy* (Homewood, Illinois: Dow Jones–Irwin, 1985).

7. Karl Albrecht, *At America's Service* (Homewood, Illinois: Dow Jones–Irwin, 1988).

8. Jan Carlzon, *Moments of Truth* (Cambridge, Massachusetts: Ballinger, 1987).

9. Albrecht, *At America's Service*.

10. Thomas J. Peters and Robert H. Waterman, Jr., *In Search of Excellence: Lessons from America's Best-Run Companies* (New York: Harper and Row, 1982).

11. Carlzon, *Moments of Truth*.

12. Albrecht, *At America's Service*.

13. Albrecht, *At America's Service*.

9.

Selecting a Technology for Communication between Health Care Providers

Improving the speed of communications with physicians, as well as the quality and quantity of important information transferred, could greatly improve physician satisfaction with the services of a health care organization. Improved communications can also benefit patients, who may be able to schedule services and receive test reports and other information more quickly and accurately.

There are a number of technologies that could be used to improve communications between health care providers, including physicians and hospitals. Improving mail communications through scheduling and referral systems that include word-processing capabilities was discussed in Chapters 4 and 5. Teleradiology links were discussed in Chapter 7.

Regional and national telephone companies and a number of other hardware and software vendors can provide information on how ordinary telephone communications could be improved to reduce delays and to allow customers to retrieve information and place orders. This includes "automated attendant" systems that allow the caller to send a call to the most appropriate department, and "voice response" systems that allow the caller to place an order by pressing a button on the phone. C. R. Hardy has described a range of such technologies to improve customer service in a managed care organization.[1]

In this chapter, several technologies that permit the transfer of information to a computer and between computers are discussed, including computer links between providers, fax transmission, digital dictation, voice mail, and voice recognition systems. The differences between the technologies that could affect the choice among them are then discussed.

To illustrate how the criteria described in Chapter 8 might be applied, a specific technology—computer links between health care providers—is then examined in detail. Although more expensive than fax, this technology has received considerable attention in articles and books as potentially one way to increase physician referrals to a hospital. It is frequently included as one option in developing a "physician bonding" program, that is, a series of activities designed to increase the loyalty of physicians and the volume of patients they refer.[2]

The choices faced by organizations that want to implement a link are presented, and the criteria described in Chapter 8 are applied to assess the desirability of this technology. Of course, the final answers will depend on the specific internal and external environment facing a particular health care organization.

Three of the cases in Part IV deal with organizations implementing a computer link. They suggest that very different systems can be developed even though a single name has been given to this technology. A careful examination of the situation facing these organizations led to the development of the criteria in Chapter 8 and many of the conclusions arrived at in this chapter.

Description of the Technologies

Hospital-to-Physician Computer Links

Hardware and software are available for linking the computers of physicians, hospitals, and other health care providers to allow the sharing of information, the scheduling of services, consultations and second opinions, and access to a range of computer programs and data bases.[3]

The simplest way to link the computers is to give users software that allows their computer to imitate, or "emulate," the terminal of the main, or "host," computer. For example, a physician's personal computer (PC) would function like a terminal connected to a hospital's IBM mainframe. Using a modem to communicate over the telephone lines, physicians could do anything in their offices that they could do in the hospital itself.

More complex systems make the software for linking computers part of the management information system of the user. A physician and staff, for example, could then move data from the hospital's billing system into the physician's billing system, without reentering the data into the physician's computer files. Further details on how computer links operate are contained later in this chapter.

Fax

Fax machines send pictures of pages over the telephone. A fax machine consists of three major components: a scanner to convert a document into a digital message (i.e., a series of zeros and ones), a fax modem to convert the digital message into audible tones that are transmitted over standard telephone lines (and to reconvert incoming tones), and a printer. The more sophisticated machines have internal memory and can receive several documents, retain them, and print them out later. Some machines allow the user to send a document to numerous other fax machines.

One of the advantages of a fax machine in comparison with a computer is that almost all fax machines sold in the United States follow what is known as the Group 3 international fax protocol. Virtually every fax machine can send a document to every other fax machine. At the relatively low resolution defined by this standard, however, a page is fuzzy but legible.

Computers can send and receive fax transmissions and provide capabilities previously available to users of computer or electronic mail. Software has been developed that can select individuals from a data base and send a fax to all of them. A fax that described a new technology useful in orthopedics could be sent to all orthopedists on a hospital's medical staff. A data base that includes the fax numbers and specialties of physicians is required. If the data are available, physicians could be selected on the basis of the zip code of their offices, their length of time on the medical staff, and their volume of admissions.

A device called a fax board can be put into a personal computer to allow it to send and receive fax transmissions. Such boards cost between $400 and $1,500. Computer files (for example, a letter in a word processor) can be converted and sent. A document that is not stored in the computer has to be entered using a device called a scanner. Some hand-held scanners can be purchased for $200–300; scanners capable of capturing a full page can cost $1,500 or more.

Uses

Since a fax machine uses ordinary telephone lines and can communicate with almost any other fax machine, it allows physicians to communicate with each other:

— General surgeons' offices use fax to move reports to referring physicians.

— Gynecologists send and receive mammogram results.

— Radiologists send gastrointestinal series results to internists.

— Physicians refer patients to specialists and surgeons and transmit patient files by fax.

Hospitals, pharmacies, nursing homes, and other health care organizations can use a fax machine[4,5] to:

— order prescriptions

— transmit lab results

— transmit special dietary or care information

— transmit insurance forms

— receive patient information from the hospital or physician

— send electrocardiogram tracings to the nurses' station or directly to a cardiologist for interpretation

— transmit accounts payable and receivable information

The use of a fax machine can help improve the productivity of staff by eliminating the hand-carrying of documents within an organization, in addition to speeding external communications.

At least two hospitals—Christian Hospitals Northeast-Northwest, St. Louis, and Memorial Hospital of South Bend (Indiana)—have paid the cost of providing fax machines to some of their physicians. Participating physicians are required to pay the phone charges.[6,7] St. Anthony's Hospital, St. Petersburg, Florida, has established a network, but has not purchased fax machines for physicians.

The Southwest Texas Methodist Hospital in San Antonio studied the impact of using a fax machine instead of pharmacy delivery aides to transmit orders to the hospital pharmacy.[8] Three nurses' stations received fax machines, while three others served as a control. Control stations averaged 82.8 minutes turnaround time per order, while floors using fax averaged 60.41 minutes, a savings of 22.39 minutes. The fax machines also increased accountability for the location of physician orders by providing confirmations of each order sent or received, and provided an exact copy of the original order to the pharmacy, as required by pharmacy law, within seconds of transmission. There were potential savings in labor costs since delivery of orders accounted for 60 percent of the time spent by pharmacy delivery aides.

Voice Communication via a Computer

Voice recognition

Voice recognition systems allow the computer to match spoken words to a known vocabulary. Once the computer knows that a spoken word matches a word stored in the computer, it can then use the computer-stored words to take a variety of actions. It can display or print the words as text. If the words are commands, it can execute them (for example, save or delete a document).[9]

A basic system with a 1,000-word vocabulary to assist in preparing reports for a radiology practice cost approximately $15,000 in 1989. A system with a 5,000-word vocabulary cost approximately $25,000.[10] These prices do not include the purchase of a personal computer (a PC/AT or compatible).

The voice recognition systems that are currently on the market have several significant limitations. They must be "trained" to understand the words of each user; each physician who wishes to use such a system to transcribe a report must repeat each word that he/she intends to use several times in order to record his/her distinct speech patterns in the computer. When a report is dictated, the computer compares the sounds to the stored vocabulary to see if there is a match. If no match is found, no word is entered into the system. Systems also require "discrete speech," i.e., that there is a pause between words. If the speaker fails to pause, the system may be unable to match the sounds to a word stored in its vocabulary.

Some prototype systems have eliminated the need for individual training and can recognize speech from many different speakers. They also can recognize continuous speech, where words are not separated by pauses. No systems with these characteristics are currently on the market.

The requirement that each speaker train the system to understand each word is a significant limitation for most health care organizations. This requires that busy radiologists or pathologists spend the time at a computer terminal repeating each word they intend to use several times. Some systems reduce the burden by storing "trigger phrases," phrases that the computer matches to individual words. A radiologist could therefore substitute the word "normal" for an entire sentence, or even paragraph, reducing the time it takes to transcribe and the time spent training the computer. The predetermined text can include "fill-ins," places where words can be inserted, such as the location and size of a tumor.

A system can be delivered with trigger phrases that are commonly used by a specialty (for example, emergency medicine, radiology, and pathology), which can then be modified by the individual physician. This represents a significant change in the way a physician dictates a report, however. The physicians must remember what phrases the words stand for, look at the computer screen as the computer displays the text that each word generates, or review the final report and edit it using the keyboard.

For a radiologist, viewing a computer screen rather than a film during dictation could be a major distraction. At least one prototype system offers a partial solution by allowing the physician to play back the full text in a synthesized voice, which would allow the physician never to take his/her eyes off the film.

Digital dictation/voice mail

The second type of technology stores spoken words in computer memory in the same way that a digital recording stores music (i.e., as a string of zeros and ones). Systems that use digital recording of spoken words are called digital dictation or voice mail systems, depending on their primary function. No attempt is made to translate the spoken words into a vocabulary understood by the computer. The words can neither be displayed as text nor serve as commands that the computer can act on.[11]

Uses

Voice recognition systems have an enormous potential for saving time and money in health care organizations. Allowing someone to talk to a computer and storing the information as text would eliminate the need to transcribe a huge quantity of information that is normally dictated, including radiology and pathology reports. Professionals would benefit greatly by being able to speak, rather than write, the large number of orders, notes, and other brief forms of communication that are not normally dictated and transcribed. This is especially true in emergency medicine departments, where physicians often have limited time to prepare reports.

Additionally, use of the computer would be greatly facilitated if professionals could use their voice to issue commands that would then be carried out by the computer. This would include making requests for the retrieval and display of information, and ordering services.

Systems that store spoken words in digital form also have a number of uses. Digital dictation systems allow referring physicians to hear the report of a radiologist, pathologist, or other consulting physician without waiting for the report to be transcribed and sent. Physicians can immediately access the report over any telephone. One system allows physicians to retrieve information entered by registered nurses on the condition of patients receiving home care services.[12]

Voice mail systems can allow a physician to store a message for retrieval by hospital staff, regardless of whether the phones are busy. Staff are alerted by the system that a message is waiting and can retrieve it. Physicians can be given voice mailboxes that store spoken messages, which they can retrieve from any phone, including a mobile cellular phone. This can supplement the traditional answering service, and eliminate lost calls and inaccurate phone messages by allowing the physician to hear the words of the caller. No research has been done on the reactions of physicians to voice mail, although studies have been done in other industries.[13]

Choosing a Technology

Fax machines or a computer link?

Fax machines have emerged as a competing technology to computer links for communication. Fax machines are cheaper than a computer, and fax transmission is very easy. A fax is also a paper document, what most clerical staff and professionals are used to handling. Physicians and their office staffs can also use fax machines to communicate with vendors, lawyers, and any other businesses that have a machine, but a computer link offers access to just the hospital and others connected to the link.

Fax does have some relative disadvantages, especially when a file of information has to be transmitted. Fax transmissions are slower because fax machines send pictures of characters, rather than the computer codes for those characters. Because of the limited internal memory and slow printers found in most fax machines, fax transmission of a patient file can tie up the telephone line for much longer than the transmission of a computer file. The scanners and printers on less expensive fax machines also produce fuzzy, if legible, documents on thermal paper that degrades in sunlight. Many people, therefore, photocopy their fax documents, adding work and expense to the process.

A fax machine also transmits illegible handwriting; computer transmission requires input into a computer. Computer communication transfers the burden of translation to the sender, rather than the receiver (although a sender can still transmit errors).

Some computer programs (for example, a scheduler) can also check for errors in incoming computer transmissions (for example, a request for a test that was just performed on a patient)—not possible with a fax transmission. Data sent by fax cannot be directly entered onto a bill or into a medical record, a capability of some practice management software tied to a computer link that can save office staff time.

These advantages of a computer link are likely to be outweighed by the low cost, ease, and familiarity of fax transmission in the eyes of some physicians and their office staffs. This will be especially true when the data available and the functions that can be performed on a computer link are limited. Sophisticated systems that allow for direct data entry onto bills and into medical records, that provide electronic claims submission, and that allow direct access by the physician to test results coming from automated lab equipment will be more competitive with fax because they offer additional benefits.

Even when a sophisticated system is in place, sending and receiving fax transmissions to perform functions that could be done with a computer link will be necessary to induce some physicians and their office staffs with a low level of interest or high level of anxiety about using a computer to participate in a program to improve communications. Although a fax machine is a combination of a microprocessor, memory, modem, and printer, it is not viewed as a computer and does not produce the anxiety that computers produce. It can also transmit handwritten notes and records that make up a substantial part of a patient's medical record without the use of a keyboard.

The danger of encouraging the use of a fax is that it may make it very difficult to justify the cost of developing the more advanced features of a computer link, for example, direct physician scheduling of services with checks for inconsistencies and errors. Fewer physicians will benefit from such features. The hospital and its medical staff could wind up with an easy-to-use, low-cost, but limited, communications system that has no capacity for expansion in the services it provides.

Voice communications?

Voice recognition systems now on the market have limited applications because of their inability to recognize many voices and continuous speech. Their primary application is likely to be in assisting individuals who produce a volume of text or whose reports are required immediately (for example, radiologists, pathologists, and emergency medicine physicians). Even here it is not clear what the benefit is to the physician, as opposed to the organization. A physician who trains and uses a voice recognition system is primarily saving the organization money by reducing the amount of transcription. If a queue would otherwise develop for transcription, time is also being saved. Accuracy is enhanced when a queue for transcription is eliminated because the physician is not required to verify the accuracy of a report when it is signed several days later.

But speed and accuracy could also be increased if the organization hired more transcriptionists. Some radiologists may still prefer voice recognition systems, however, because they can eliminate the time spent correcting errors in a report prepared by a transcriptionist. Since voice recognition systems now cost $15,000–25,000, excluding a computer (which would cost about $3,000–5,000 more), they are attractive investments to the organization when compared to the hiring of transcriptionists. The challenge will be to convince physicians that they also benefit by changing the way they practice.

Digital dictation and voice mail is the appropriate alternative to voice recognition systems when a large number of people need to transmit smaller amounts of information. Digital dictation and voice mail systems are not an alternative to fax machines and computer links because they do not transmit documents and data unless they are spoken, which would result in errors.

They can be useful supplements, however. They can allow staff to reach a physician where no fax machine or computer is available. They allow physicians to communicate to their offices and the hospital in similar situations. They also provide a stored record of what the physician said, increasing accountability.

Digital dictation and voice mail may, however, meet some of the same resistance as answering machines: they will be viewed by some people as impersonal and unresponsive. A physician who receives a digitally stored message rather than a personal phone call may feel that the caller did not have the interest or respect to pursue the physician and deliver the message personally. Many physicians are also interested in immediate resolution of a problem. Leaving a voice message can be useful in stating problems but does not offer the potential for immediate resolution offered by a conversation.

Health care organizations should also be concerned about the implicit promise of service made by establishing these systems. A physician who knows that digitally stored reports are available as soon as they are spoken will expect them faster. A physician who leaves a voice message about a problem may assume that it will be immediately resolved. The organization needs to understand the expectations by continually talking with the medical staff and either lowering (through education—either personal or by newsletters and other written communications) or meeting those expectations. Otherwise, physician dissatisfaction may be the end result.

Physician-to-Hospital Computer Links

New systems for linking the computers of health care providers are continually being introduced. This chapter will not attempt to compare and evaluate the current systems because such descriptions and evaluations would be out-of-date very quickly. Instead, we will describe the choices available to buyers and the potential of systems to enhance services to physicians and patients.

Choices for Developers

Systems differ depending on the answers given by their developers to the following questions:

— Do we want a computer network or a link between computers that allows data to be examined and transferred?

— Should the link require connection to a single central computer, or allow users' computers to connect directly with each other?

— What data should be available to those who use the link?

— Should the link be an integrated part of each user's management computer system?

— How much support do we want to give to clinical decision making?

Network or link?

Most of the systems now on the market allow the user to examine and transfer certain data. They do not allow the sharing of hardware or access to data bases stored on many computers in the system. The term *computer link* will be used in this chapter to refer to such systems.

A computer link between physicians and a hospital allows physicians access to a hospital's computer and to some of its data bases. Data can be examined and transferred to the physician's computer. Information can also be sent by the physician to the hospital.

A computer *network* would allow all users access to some files on many computers in the network and could allow the sharing of peripherals such as printers. Even memory could be shared if a particular user did not have enough. A hospital participating in a computer network would then be able to access a physician's billing or other files (depending on prior agreements) and physicians would be able to use the printers and memory of the hospital's (or other physicians') computer for tasks such as billing.

Computer networks require a higher level of cooperation and trust, as well as more advanced security systems to block unauthorized access to data that would violate patient and physician confidentiality. A network may also be viewed as undesirable because it permits the sharing of information that could influence negotiations over services and fees between physicians and hospitals.

The software required to operate a network is also more expensive, and a network requires more (and more expensive) staff or consultants. It is therefore not surprising that most systems are computer links, rather than networks.

Central computer?

Some systems allow for communications between any computers without using a central host computer. This would allow, for example, two physicians to exchange data without using a central hospital computer. Other systems allow communication only through a central computer.

Allowing communication between any computers is helpful when the available central computer is overworked or out-of-date, when there are concerns about allowing outside users access to the central computer, or where the sponsor wishes to establish links in incremental steps. It is also useful when users are concerned that the operators of the central computer will use their knowledge of the flow of information to their own advantage.

For example, a hospital may wish to establish a link to a single computer system in the hospital (for example, lab or radiology), but not the hospital's central computer. This could be for security reasons—some hospital data-processing managers are very concerned about unauthorized parties gaining access to a hospital's computer over the telephone—or because the hospital's computer has reached maximum capacity or is out-of-date. By developing a system that allows communication between any computers in the system, the hospital can encourage communications with physicians without waiting for replacement or upgrading of its central computer, or advances in computer security. The lab or radiology system becomes one of the computers in the system, and others can be added, including any new central computer that is acquired.

Physicians may prefer that the hospital computer not be the central node in a system out of concern that their communications with other physicians, as well as billing and patient data sent to insurance companies over the system, might be accessed by hospital staff and somehow used to their disadvantage in negotiations with the hospital.

Some physicians will emphatically reject any connection between the computer they use for patient records, billing, and accounting, and the hospital's computer. A negative and emotional reaction can be based on one or more factors.

One factor may be a misunderstanding of the technical capabilities of the system. Some physicians believe that the hospital will be able to transfer data from their computer to the hospital without their knowledge or consent. This is not true in almost all cases, although some software vendors do use software that allows a service representative to solve problems without a visit to the site by operating the computer from a central location. Physicians concerned about the possibility of unauthorized transfer must be educated about the technical capabilities of the system being installed. In some cases, the system being installed should be modified to make an upload, or transfer, of certain files impossible. The system described in the Cleveland Clinic case (Chapter 11) is a "store-and-forward" system, that is, messages are stored in one computer and then forwarded to the other when the central computer is available. The central computer never accesses a data base in the remote computer, so nothing can be transferred from those data bases.

Another factor may be a concern that hospital staff will have their "nose in my books." This is a real concern, even if the transfer of files is made impossible, when hospital staff or a firm working for the hospital install a practice management system for the physician. Installation and maintenance of an accounting and patient billing component will require access to the physician's financial records. If physicians are concerned, other ways of providing a practice management system can be arranged. For example,

Samaritan Health Services (see Chapter 12) offers physicians information about a number of vendors of practice management software who have agreed to support the link. Physicians made the choice and pay for the software themselves, reducing the concern that the vendor is working for the hospital. No hospital staff are involved in installation and maintenance.

A third factor may be a concern that the hospital is attempting to infringe on the physician's independence. A more general concern is that the hospital is moving in the direction of controlling information that is critical to the physician's independence and livelihood. Hospitals that offer to install practice management systems and use hospital data to speed up claims processing, and to forward claims for electronic processing, might face this charge. Some physicians feel that control of their practice is already being lost to government, insurance companies, and review organizations, all of whom are collecting and using data on the physician in ways that are threatening to the physician's independence. The hospital that offers an array of new information services—even though the intent is to help the physician—may find itself lumped with "the enemy."

There are a range of possible solutions to these problems. Physicians are frequently most influenced by their peers, so support of the new system by respected physicians is essential. Education about the technology is also important. Finally, the hospital faced with significant opposition for the reasons mentioned above may wish to distance itself from the provision of many services. Like Samaritan Health Services, they may screen vendors and offer information about them to physicians, but not sell or service a practice management system or hardware. By offering only to facilitate the transfer of hospital data to the physician, physician opposition may be reduced.

What data should be available?

Major considerations in developing a link or network are what data bases will be accessible and what a user will be allowed to do that changes a data base. The most conservative strategy is to establish a data base separate from all others that can be accessed from a remote site. A remote user would not be able to change anything in that data base. A less conservative strategy would allow a user to examine the actual data base in day-to-day use, but not change anything. Finally, the user could be treated as equivalent to the organization's own staff and be allowed to make changes in the data base where appropriate.

Some hospitals, concerned about unauthorized access to data bases, have developed systems where physicians can only access data bases specifically designed for them. Changes in these data bases would have no effect on hospital operations. Other hospitals have allowed access to the information systems of hospital departments, such as radiology or lab, to allow physicians to look at schedules and test results without changing any data. A request for a service could be entered, for example, but the physician's office could not enter an appointment in the scheduling system. A confirmation of an appointment is sent to the physician's office at a later time. A third possibility would be to allow the physician's office to actually use a hospital's computer system to request services, schedule appointments, and enter data from the physician's office directly into the hospital's billing and medical records systems. So, in addition to the decision on hardware and software, a major decision that a hospital must make, therefore, is what it will allow a physician to do, based on its understanding of physician needs and desires and its own concerns about the integrity of its data bases and confidentiality.

Concerns about patient and physician confidentiality, as well as unauthorized tampering with hospital data, have therefore led to a wide variation in the data that flows to and from the hospital's computer. The information that flows *from* the hospital can include:

— data needed to complete patient bills (including discharge diagnoses, discharge abstracts, and operative summaries), allowing faster billing and avoiding reentry of the data

— results of tests done and records of medications administered

— up-to-date rounds reports on inpatients

— responses to requests for consultations

— general requests for information, such as whether the physician has completed the chart review and attestations required for Medicare billing

— responses to requests for information from data bases stored or accessed through the hospital, such as information on drug combinations that are contraindicated

The information that flows *to* the hospital can include:

— requests to schedule services at the hospital, including lab, radiology, and other ancillary services

— patient histories and the results of physicals

— admitting orders and information for inpatient preadmission forms

— test results, for example, for stress ECGs that the physician wants evaluated

— patient bills, if the hospital has agreed to submit them electronically or manages the physician's accounting and receivables system

— queries and other commands necessary to receive the data and information listed above from the hospital

Systems integration?

Any computer system is easier to use when the commands and procedures that are involved are simple and similar to those in other computer programs. An important decision in developing a provider link is how much time and money should be spent to create commands and procedures (i.e., a user interface) that make it easier to learn and use the link.

A computer program could be used that permits a remote computer to emulate a terminal used on the host computer. An IBM PC would then function as if it were a Digital Equipment Company VAX or IBM mainframe terminal. Such "terminal emulation" software requires that the person using the link understand the commands necessary to use the host computer. Instead of entering the commands used to operate the PC, the user would enter the commands appropriate for the host computer. Other systems use a program called a "front-end processor" that can convert a series of commands into the language needed by the host computer.

If the host computer uses a difficult (to understand and learn) computer language, terminal emulation could result in considerable frustration. A front-end processor offers another advantage if the same one is used to control word processing, accounting, and other office functions. Office staff only have to learn one set of commands in order to use all the programs.

However, terminal emulation software is less expensive than a front-end processor, since thousands of users will want to access and emulate a terminal of the popular mainframe and minicomputer models. Selecting a single front-end processor to give to all users of the link would provide some help, but the commands would still not be the same as those used by the individual word processors and other software currently in use. The most expensive strategy would be to create a front-end processor that has commands and procedures similar to each of the accounting, medical records, and word-processing packages in use.

A less expensive alternative is to provide or sell a package of programs for accounting, billing, and word processing and include software for linking computers that has the same user interface. Data transfer between computers then becomes another choice on the menu of options, rather than a special function that requires knowledge of another computer system and its language. Individuals who do not want the package can be given or sold just the program for establishing the link to use by itself.

Integrating the software for linking computers into a larger package offers other advantages. Programs can be written that put transferred data directly into billing and medical records forms without any additional typing. Patient registration can be completed without asking patients for information already provided to the hospital and reentering it into the computer. Someone who uses just the software for establishing the link would have to (1) transfer the data and then (2) either reenter the data into a form or create a computer program to do so.

To use such an integrated product, however, a user would have to switch from their existing software, for example, for accounting and billing. If the existing system was unsatisfactory, the effort and problems involved in the change might be justified. If the user was generally pleased with the existing system, the costs of changing would have to be compared with the benefits of integration, for example, reduced clerical time and faster billing.

One way to reduce the reluctance of the user to switch is to provide consulting and other services. However, this could slow the growth in the number of users if trained staff are not available. A hospital that wanted to assist physicians in changing to a new (or their first) computer-based accounting and finance system would have to hire and train specialists in accounting and staff training. This could slow network development and would have to be justified by greater physician loyalty to a system that would be difficult to abandon once installed, by the profits made from systems sales and maintenance, or by both.

Support for clinical decision making?

Although many current systems emphasize administrative functions, a wide range of computer-based tools useful in clinical decision making continues to appear. Data bases are available that contain abstracts of medical books and journals (which could be searched for relevant studies) as well as the contents of reference books such as the *Physician's Desk Reference* (which lists all available drugs and when they should and should not be used). New computer programs are constantly being written that assist physicians in making diagnoses or decisions about treatment.

The potential exists to create an information source that is routinely used by the physician, rather than by the physician's office staff. Presumably, such a system would be viewed by the physician as valuable and difficult to give up in favor of a competing computer system.

Some factors that need to be considered are whether a clinically oriented system would be attractive to, and widely used by, physicians. One research study on physician use of computers suggests that computer use is directly related to whether the physician has a peer group currently using computers.[14] The existence of a peer group actively using computers to assist in clinical decision making may be an important factor in the success of a clinically oriented system.

The ability to quantify the benefits of a clinically oriented system may also determine its success. It is easier to quantify the impact of a link on the cost of administrative functions than the contribution it makes to clinical decisions. Because the physician is the primary user, however, and can directly judge the importance of the clinical information received, rigorous studies of the cost and benefits of a system may be less important.

The IMS 2000™ system being used by the Cleveland Clinic (described in Chapter 11) is an example of another possibility. It offers the physician both access to specialized information and the ability to perform medical tests that generate revenue. The physician, therefore, has both a financial and professional interest in acquiring and operating the system.

For whatever reasons, current systems provide tools for clinical decision making as supplementary, rather than central, elements of the package of services.

Potential for Enhancing Services

Interviews with users and developers, product marketing literature, and a review of the professional literature suggest that the objective of physician-to-hospital computer links are to:

— increase the use of hospital services

— reward the physician for current and future loyalty to the hospital, that is, use of hospital services

— increase the costs of using competing services

— improve compliance with hospital requirements, for example, submission of data needed for billing and regulatory requirements

— improve the practice of medicine

Whether the technology can accomplish these objectives will be critically examined later. First, it is important to understand the logic that is used in seeing a computer link as being capable of achieving these objectives. The critical assumptions are

— physicians will value faster and easier access to hospital information and services for their staff and patients

— the value added is high enough to convince a physician to use a hospital's service instead of a competitor's

— the hospital will improve its data collection by having access to physician data

— physicians will frequently use reference data bases and clinical decision-making software in their medical practices

A physician's office would become like a travel agency. A computer terminal linked to the supplier—a hospital rather than airlines—would become an indispensable means of carrying out business. If removed, it would result in considerable inconvenience to the physician. The physician would be unlikely to change to a competing computer system because of the high value added of the one being used and the cost in time and errors of teaching the staff to use it. A second analogy—applicable to a second generation of systems—is that such systems become electronic libraries of essential information for practicing medicine. Again, the physician would be unwilling to do without the system or to use a competing system because of the value lost and the cost of switching in time and errors made.

The travel agency analogy is not entirely appropriate. The travel agent uses the computer to perform the core element of the service. Current systems for physicians assist in functions that—although important—are not why patients come to the physician. Patients come not to be billed or to have medical information quickly and accurately transferred, but to receive medical services and get well. A major question facing sponsors of these systems is whether they should increase their value for the practice of medicine, or continue to enhance their capabilities for assisting in billing and other administrative functions.

An article in the *Annals of Internal Medicine* described a survey of 625 office-based physicians and 100 physician "opinion leaders." Less than one in three physicians reported searching the medical literature themselves for information; two in three claimed the volume of literature was unmanageable.[15] Although a computer link could provide physicians with access to data bases containing the medical literature (for example, the National Library of Medicine's MEDLINE system), they will not solve the problem physicians have reading the large number of studies that are often identified or assessing their value. Although the library analogy may be appropriate, this service enhancement may not be highly valued until the medical profession develops a way of summarizing and critiquing the literature concerning a particular problem.

Are the Criteria Met?

Before a commitment is made to acquire or enhance a computer link, the criteria described in Chapter 8 need to be applied. The answers will depend on the specific system under consideration, the objectives and capabilities of the sponsoring organization, and the needs and desires of physicians and patients. This section cannot provide a final answer to the questions raised. What follows are some insights gained from studying systems now in place.

Who benefits?

1. Who will primarily benefit?   Who primarily benefits will depend on the capabilities of the system. The primary benefits of systems that stress the transmission of billing information and the scheduling of hospital procedures go to the physician's office staff. If the staff is overworked, the benefit to the physician may be a savings in salaries and wages that results from not having to hire additional staff. If the staff is not overworked, then the benefit to the physician is less tangible—staff morale. If the system is enhanced to include electronic claims submission, then improved cash flow could provide a tangible benefit directly to the physician.

Note that systems designed to be used by office staff are likely to be perceived as valuable by the physician to the extent that the results are tracked and presented to the physician. On the other hand, systems that are used by the physician, for example, to retrieve data on treatment protocols, provide benefits that are directly visible to the physician.

Will utilization be affected?

2. *What role do they play in determining if your services are used?* There may be several individuals involved in deciding where a patient will receive services. A computer link that primarily benefits the office staff could be particularly important when the nurse/receptionist has a role in deciding where a patient goes. This sometimes occurs for routine lab and radiology services, where the physician may find several providers acceptable and leaves it to the office staff and patient to decide who can "fit the patient in." A call by the office staff then results in the scheduling of the patient with one provider as opposed to another.

In the case of other services—for example, admission for surgery—the office staff may play no role at all. The physician may have the major role in making a decision. Finally, there are services where patients desire to select a provider based on their own criteria. These may include routine mammography services, the selection of an obstetrician, a place to give birth, or a pediatrician.

For the computer link to have an effect on referrals, it must offer additional value to the individual primarily responsible for making the decision. The organization sponsoring the network needs to specify the services or procedures where an increase in utilization is most desired and then examine who primarily makes the decision. The system could be particularly effective, for example, in affecting the use of routine ancillary services such as lab and radiology, where the ability to quickly schedule and get back the results is perceived as valuable by office staff and physicians. On the other hand, it may have little effect on the use of surgical services, where physicians' tastes and preferences in operating room staff and equipment are far more important than the speed with which the patient is scheduled.

Another approach would be to target specific physicians and use a package of computer-based services as an enticement. Borgess Medical Center carried out an analysis of the demographic and economic characteristics of the population in 15 surrounding counties. Management and consultants identified selected zip codes where the population was relatively affluent and well insured. The primary care physicians serving those zip codes were identified, and an offer of a free computer with printers and software was then made to them, as well as to selected staff specialists. Borgess recognized that 65 percent of its patients come from primary care physicians, and that a core of 110 primary care physicians made most referrals in its market area.[16] Borgess chose to focus on a group of physicians rather than a specific service since these physicians use a wide range of hospital services. Although no one computer-based service might boost utilization, a rich package of free services was expected to increase use of the medical center.

3. What are the expected benefits? How large will they be? Scheduling and the receipt of results offer savings in time; electronic claims submission offers savings in money, since additional cash can be invested. It is important to specify to the provider to be served just what the benefits of a particular system are and quantify how large they may be.

Note that some time savings, in fact, add little value to the service being offered. If physicians have traditionally asked patients to call the hospital and schedule a test themselves, then the time savings of remote scheduling do not represent a benefit to the physician unless it can be linked to both higher consumer satisfaction and increased patient loyalty to the physician. Patient expectations of the physician are critically important because they may not see the physician as responsible for any difficulty in scheduling a test.

Another example is test results. If the physician intends to act quickly, then fast results are important. If, however, the physician has a set time for seeing the patient, the results could arrive one day or five days before the appointment. The difference is not meaningful to the physician or the patient. Again, it is important to ask for which service a savings in time, because it will be perceived by the patient, physician, or both as a benefit, is important.

Computer networks can create new services, for example, a second reading, or "overread," of a pulmonary function test (see the Cleveland Clinic case in Chapter 11). The physician's or patient's desire for the service, rather than the computer link, is the issue.

4. Are benefits of this magnitude **known** *to be important in the decision to use your services?* The preceding discussion raises questions rather than answering them. An organization considering the development of a computer link needs to confirm who benefits, by how much, in what ways, and whether it makes a difference in service utilization.

Since the investment in this technology is large, answers confirmed by market research are essential. This may be done by surveys that ask about attitudes, beliefs, and probable behavior, or by pilot studies with physicians, patients, and services where an increase in service volume (or no loss in market share) is desired.

5. Could providing the benefits differentiate you from competitors or reduce their competitive advantage?   The computer link will differentiate a provider from competitors; the question is whether the value added by the link is large enough to create a competitive advantage or reduce one held by a competitor. Meaningful differentiation is the issue, that is, differentiation that results in a change in the behavior of physicians and patients.

Is the proposed use ethical and legal?

6. Will the proposed program be viewed as unethical?   The transfer of information between physicians and hospitals is a routine part of the process of delivering health services that, in itself, raises no ethical issues as long as the norms for confidentiality of information are followed. The ethical issues in the development of a hospital-to-physician computer link are:

1. Who will pay the cost of the resources that are required, including hardware, software, and support services such as maintenance, training, and the development of the data bases required?

2. What will the physician be asked to do, if anything, in return for participation?

The issue of cost sharing is often decided by legal requirements, but managers should be sensitive to the ethical arguments. Members of the board, managers, staff, clinicians, and external groups are likely to object to the hospital providing free goods and services to physicians. Some physicians will, however, argue that solving the hospital's problems (for example, with the telephone system) should not cost physicians anything. It will be necessary to demonstrate the benefits to the physicians to deal with this issue, although some physicians will still refuse to participate if they have to pay.

A more difficult question is the extent to which the organization can ethically subsidize an activity that could potentially improve patient care. Some subsidy could be viewed as ethical if health care services are likely to be of higher quality because information was transferred more quickly, accurately, and completely. The exact proportion of the total cost that should be borne by the hospital is open to debate.

Some hospitals avoid this issue by providing no cash subsidy. To reduce the cost to physicians, they use the hospital's ability to negotiate discounts or lease arrangements to benefit the physician who wishes to purchase hardware and software. However, the hospital usually bears entirely the cost of altering its own software and developing the data bases that will be used by the link. Only a part of this is an incremental cost, which is then justified on the basis of benefits to the hospital and patients.

Cash payments to assist physicians in acquiring hardware and software are the most controversial since a judgment must be made on the extent to which the physician personally benefits from the link, and no mathematical formula exists for determining this. The Cleveland Clinic (see Chapter 11) asked physicians to pay one-third (or $35 per month in 1989) of the cost of a basic workstation, software for communications and support, and maintenance. Physicians also had to lease a dedicated telephone line for $35 per month. Vassar Brothers Hospital lent hardware and software to physicians for the pilot test (which Samaritan Health Services also did) while the board considered how to deal with the pricing issue. Samaritan Health Services offered to provide physicians with free communications software and to provide hardware for $600 per year for five years (the estimated cost of hardware and software was $3,100 per site). Because of the difficulty of making judgments about what level of subsidy is ethical, the final decision is often made on the basis of the advice of legal counsel.

The second issue is what physicians will be asked to do, if anything, in return for participation. It is widely considered unethical (and certainly illegal when Medicare patients are involved) to require that physicians refer any of their patients to the hospital. Unspoken expectations are the major issue. Intent is used as one ethical test. If the hospital establishes the program with the intent of affecting the volume of referrals, it may be viewed as unethical regardless of what other benefits are produced. This would make a program unethical in which any physician on the medical staff, regardless of their volume of referrals, is offered subsidized hardware and software. The argument here is that the hospital should not be attempting to influence physicians to make decisions on any other grounds than the patient's welfare. Of course, it could also be argued that the program would be unethical if it had this effect, regardless of what the hospital's intent was. Again, the advice of legal counsel resolves this ethical issue in many cases. The issue of what to require physicians to do is usually settled by establishing no requirements for participation.

However, the link may be marketed to physicians who could benefit the hospital by changing their referral patterns or who are expected to provide more referrals within the next few years (for example, younger physicians who have just entered the community). The Cleveland Clinic and Samaritan Health Services adopted this policy. For the pilot phase, both Samaritan Health Services and Vassar Brothers also included physicians and groups who provided a large number or high proportion of their inpatient admissions to the hospital.

7. Is the proposed program legal? Current federal Medicare and Medicaid fraud and abuse laws do not currently forbid computer links intended to encourage hospital admissions.[17] A number of attorneys recommend that hospitals follow these guidelines in establishing a program:[18]

— The program should be available to all members of the medical staff, not just physicians who admit a large number of patients.

— Physicians should be required to contribute financially to the system's cost.

— Administrators should be able to document how the system contributes to the overall quality of patient care.

It is important to note, however, that the federal government has not defined any "safe harbors," that is, programs that would be viewed as automatically legal, where the provision of goods and services to physicians is concerned. Following the guidelines listed above does not ensure that the link will be viewed as legal under federal fraud and abuse laws, state antikickback laws, or IRS regulations concerning what activities a tax-exempt organization can engage in and not endanger its tax-exempt status.

Can you sustain the competitive advantage?

8. How easy will it be for competitors to implement the technology and reduce any competitive advantage?   The technology for establishing a computer link is easy to obtain. Although an exclusive right to develop a particular system in a geographic area might be obtained from a vendor, there are alternative systems that can establish a computer link available.

This suggests that a *sustainable* competitive advantage will have to be achieved by offering services through the link that are difficult to imitate. These services should act as barriers to entry for competitors and result in high switching costs for patients and physicians.

One promising service is consultations for diagnosis and treatment using highly valued physicians whose services are difficult to obtain. The Cleveland Clinic's program of "overreads" for pulmonary function tests is an example.

Another approach is to make the link a part of a practice management system whose replacement would require considerable time and effort by the physician's staff. This strategy may lead, however, to slower growth in the network since some physicians may not be in the market for a change or installation of a major system, and those who are will require considerable help from the sponsoring organization.

The Michigan Health Care Network established by Borgess Medical Center provided a select group of physicians with a personal computer on indefinite loan and software for word processing, automatic patient billing and insurance claims processing, computerized collections reporting, and record keeping. The system allowed physicians in the network to schedule appointments with each other or to preregister patients at the hospital for tests or admissions. Experienced practice management consultants were promised to help physicians with their daily business problems. Borgess hoped that 36 would sign up in the first year; in fact, over 100 signed up in the first three months alone.[19] The physicians who use the network for all their administrative functions face high switching costs if they decide to switch. To fuel rapid growth, however, Borgess incurred $1.7 million in start-up costs. Borgess' consultants recommend budgeting $10,000 per physician practice for start-up costs, and an annual outlay of $1.5 to 4 million. Borgess' management attributed 100–200 incremental admissions per month (in 1986) to the network.

Borgess had attempted to achieve high growth rates, high switching costs, and high payoffs in hospital admissions through a high-cost strategy of implementing a more complex link at no cost to the participating physician. St. Luke's Hospital in Milwaukee, Wisconsin, took a less expensive course. Participating physicians had to buy their own hardware and pay for the software, but at a discount that gave them both AnnsonLink™ ($4,495 retail in 1986) and Doctor's Office Manager II ($3,500 retail in 1986) for less than $3,500.[20]

The question facing hospitals is whether the slower growth in the network that can be expected when physicians share a substantial part of the cost also results in fewer admissions and higher market penetration for competing links.

*9. Is being **first** to use the technology and offer its benefits likely to lead to consumer loyalty, high switching costs for consumers, or both?*   In and of itself, being first to market is unlikely to lead to high consumer loyalty or high switching costs. It is the value of the service being offered and the difficulty competitors would have in producing equal or higher value that are critical.

For example, distributing computers and terminal emulation software— the fastest way to establish a simple link—may not result in a service that is either highly valued or unique. A competitor can easily distribute terminal emulation software for its computer that can be used on the same machine. Being second to market becomes cheaper.

The computer link must be more complex and offer services with a higher value before early entry becomes a strategic advantage. If the computer link is part of a practice management system, then being first *is* critical because of the high switching costs entailed if a physician's office switches accounting, billing, and medical records systems, for example.

Evaluation

10. What is the relationship between cost and expected benefits?   It has been stressed several times in this discussion that the specific services or procedures where increased use is desired must be identified. The net revenue per unit should then be determined based on past utilization. The remaining question is then how much utilization is likely to increase. This could be estimated using survey questionnaires that focused on identifying current barriers to use that might be eliminated by using the network.

Suppose, for example, that a quick survey of a physician's office staff discloses that staff cannot reach a hospital lab to schedule an appointment because the line is busy at least once a day. The result is that an average of one patient per day is referred to a private lab. If the average net revenue for the lab tests most frequently requested is $10, then the resulting loss in income is $200 or more per month. On this basis alone, an investment by a hospital in hardware and software of $100 per month can be justified.

If, on the other hand, the service is inpatient surgery and the physician does not have admitting privileges elsewhere, the net revenue obtained as a result of the link may be zero. The investment would then have to be justified on the basis of greater physician loyalty or patient satisfaction.

If the sponsoring hospital is faced with competition from a freestanding surgery center, it may use the link to reverse an image of poor service among physicians and patients. Evaluation of the impact on net revenue of the network itself is more difficult, however. One possibility is to offer the network to one group of physicians and compare their behavior with other groups. Such experiments are difficult to carry out in practice, however, since both groups must have similar alternative services available and be matched on their characteristics (for example, stage of career, specialty).

The Management Services Division of Baxter Healthcare Corporation conducted such a study for Little Company of Mary Hospital in Evergreen Park, Illinois, in 1987.[21] The revenue generated for the hospital by a group of linked physicians was compared with three control groups. The growth in revenue between 1984 and 1986 was found to be 14 percent higher in the linked group. The range was from 20 percent for family practice physicians to 10 percent for surgeons, with internists' revenues higher by 15 percent and pediatricians' by 16 percent. Baxter estimates that the increased use of the hospital by linked physicians is resulting in $4 million in additional annual revenue.

The evaluation included interviews with physicians' office managers, 72 percent of whom felt the link increased revenues for the practice. Interviews with physicians showed that 95 percent would recommend the system to nonlinked physicians; 92 percent said that they are more likely to send patients to the hospital; 90 percent said that they experience improved cash flow; 90 percent said that their offices are more productive; and 81 percent believed that the system improves quality of care.

Increased revenue to the sponsor as a result of greater service use is only one benefit of a computer link. The type of research that has to be carried out after a link is implemented will depend on the package of services that is offered. Some services could generate fees from physicians, such as electronic claims submission and practice management services. The profits for the hospital are easily calculated. The benefits from faster and more accurate transmission of data are more difficult to measure. If hospital claims are filed faster and rejected less frequently, however, the financial results can be significant.

11. Can you (or the vendor) put in place a system for continuous monitoring of changes in service volume? Does it question customers about the importance of the benefits provided? Any computer link put in place should be able to track activity over the system by physician. This would include the number of services ordered, results requested, and other services. These should be tracked over time in management reports and compared with the period prior to implementation of the link. This information will suggest which services are highly valued. Such a series of reports should be produced on demand by the system software, rather than requiring extensive data manipulation or difficult file transfer to allow report-writing software to be used.

The vendor should be able to provide assistance in assessing system performance through surveys of providers or other means. This will allow the opportunity to determine why a service is or is not being utilized. Is it difficult for staff to learn and use with vendor support? Is a physician not really interested in using a data base on the system?

Systems that do not have such monitoring and vendors who cannot provide support in evaluation are clearly less desirable.

12. Will a system be put in place that monitors the behavioral impact of the technology on staff, patients, and physicians? If the computer link is successful, it is likely to result in competition. Competition can best be met through an understanding of what patients and physicians want and how they behave when they use a system. By monitoring how behavior changes, the sponsoring organization can both help make the current system more effective and look for innovations that could help it sustain a competitive advantage.

For example, it is a widely held belief that physicians themselves will not touch a computer, especially one that is used primarily for business functions. A system that monitors who is using the computer by looking at the passwords entered and the types of requests made can question this assumption and lead to innovations. If it is discovered, for example, that a particular physician makes frequent use of data bases containing medical journal abstracts, that physician could be offered instruction in search strategies or the latest version of software for searching the medical literature.

Physicians may not accept the computer for certain functions. As one physician noted, "Collegiality and good care still necessitate a chatty telephone conversation to fill in case background."[22]

A computer link lacks some important characteristics of a face-to-face encounter. The affective element is missing—the look of surprise, disappointment, or frustration. Even in a telephone call, it is possible to have some understanding of what the caller wants, apart from the words being said, by listening to the tone of voice, inflection, and phrasing of sentences.

Just as important is the transmission in face-to-face and telephone encounters of information on what physicians' and patients' needs and wants are, which may never be typed into the computer. Some mechanism must exist for collecting this important information in order to allow the sponsoring organization to remain innovative in its services. The computer link should not lock the organization into its current services and administrative procedures.

Any system for monitoring the behavior of people on computer networks should include both the routine collection of quantitative data on use of the system, and formal and informal interviews of the users. Again, a vendor should be able to provide support for both approaches.

Implementation

13. Is anyone in your organization responsible and accountable for service quality? Do they have the authority to institute change?   Before implementing a computer link, it is important to recognize that it will raise the expectations of patients and physicians regarding the quantity of information they will be able to access, the speed with which they will access the information, and the response time of the organization.

Failing to meet these expectations will result in a decrease, rather than increase, in physician and patient satisfaction. For example, a physician who orders a lab test for a patient on a Monday and knows that the results will be available over a computer link as soon as they leave the machine (through a direct link or interface to the computer) will have higher expectations concerning the speed with which the results will be available. Previously, when the results came by mail, the physician might assume that the mails were slow and not blame the hospital. Since the only factor determining when the results are ready is how soon the sample is put in the machine, the physician's expectations may be higher. The hospital that does not recognize this and fails to change behavior in the lab may get worse, rather than better, evaluations.

As this suggests, a computer link can only be a part of a strategy to improve service. The performance of the organization must also change, and this requires a commitment that goes beyond the purchase of hardware and software. If no one in the organization is responsible and accountable for service quality, or has the authority to institute change, it may be a good idea not to establish a computer link that allows physicians and patients to interact with the sponsoring organization on a real-time, interactive basis.

Pamela Hanlon and Andrew Kaskiw note that one of the key factors in the development of unsuccessful networks is "allowing the hospital's system implementation schedule to determine the timing of the implementation of a network strategy."[23] By allowing the hospital to remain internally oriented, management can significantly reduce the benefits of this strategy.

14. Do the responsible parties have the knowledge, willingness, and skills to acquire and install the technology?   Many hospitals have computer systems oriented to performing transactions such as billing. The maintenance of a computer link whose major purpose is real-time, interactive service to physicians and patients may require new technical skills and also a change in attitude. The users are not the employees of the hospital and will not understand or accept that the organization has other priorities.

Finding any additional technical skills is probably the easiest problem, although the managers of a sponsoring organization should be wary of statements that the system "in theory" or "in concept" does not require additional skills. Vendor support is essential, and this means contractual guarantees of training and service.

The willingness of technical staff to change their behavior is another matter, requiring continual restatement by top management of their support for the system and the offer of reasonable resources to make the computer link work.

15. Will your organization commit the resources to train and motivate front-line people (for example, nurses) to use and support the technology?   A computer link is not merely a technical innovation, but a commitment to service that can raise physician and patient expectations. If front-line people are not ready to provide that service, the benefits of the link will not be realized.

Some computer links will require no additional work for front-line personnel. Others will require that they take action faster. For example, the expectation of physicians may be that the availability of a hospital bed will be confirmed faster over a computer link. Admissions staff will have to recognize that and respond faster to requests. They can view this as onerous or an opportunity, depending on their level of motivation and whether the computer system they use poses no obstacles. Again, technology is only part of the answer.

16. Is the use of technology part of a larger effort to make service quality a superordinate goal of the organization?   As this discussion has stressed, a computer link is a part—and only a part—of a program to improve service quality. It could result in a decrease in physician and patient satisfaction if it is not part of a larger effort to improve service quality. The promise offered by a computer link is that front-line staff will have a better way to communicate with physicians and patients than overloaded telephone systems, slow mails, and computer systems that talk in obscure languages. The technology could, however, result in communicating that the organization has failed to provide a high level of service, and communicating it faster. The end result will depend on whether a much larger effort to improve service is succeeding. A computer link can only do part of the job.

A Final Word

A computer link is a service rather than a piece of technology. It is impossible, therefore, to say that computer links per se are either a good or bad investment. The market for this service needs to be studied, a service package designed, a high-quality service must be consistently delivered, and the results continually evaluated. As the examples in this chapter show, the results can be positive and produce a return on the investment made. The technology utilized also offers the potential for improving the clinical quality of health services that is just beginning to be explored.

Notes

1. C. Hardy, "Voice Processing in Managed Care," *Journal of Ambulatory Care Management* 12, no. 4 (November 1989): 17.
2. Douglas McKell and John Wire, "Physician-Hospital Computer Systems" in Stephen Valentine, ed., *Physician Bonding: Developing a Successful Hospital Program* (Rockville, Maryland: Aspen Publishers, 1989).
3. Jane Green, "The Role of Information Systems in the Hospital-Physician Relationship," *Topics in Health Care Financing* 14, no. 2 (Winter 1987): 9–16.
4. Daphne Woods, "When Seconds Count, Delta Medical Center Counts on Fax Machines," *Healthcare Computing and Communications* (November 1987): 14.
5. Loren Yamamoto and Robert Wiebe, "Improving Medical Communication with Facsimile (Fax) Transmission," *American Journal of Emergency Medicine* 7, no. 2 (March 1988): 203–8.
6. Linda Perry, "Fax Machines Link Physicians to Hospitals," *Modern Healthcare* (August 18, 1989): 62.
7. Mary Koska, "Hospital/Physician Fax Networks: Plan Ahead for Success," *Hospitals* 64, no. 4 (February 20, 1990): 75.

8. Yolanda Villarreal, "How Fax Can Cut Drug Order and Delivery Time," *Hospital Pharmacist Report* (April 1988): 13.
9. Peter Cohen, "Voice Entry in the Lab," *Computers in Healthcare* 11, no. 3 (1990): 33–36.
10. India Smith, "Voice Recognition Systems: Current Status," *Applied Radiology* (April 1989): 23.
11. Howard Rothman, "Voice Messaging Basics: Speaking Frankly," *Modern Office Technology* 34 (July 1989): 87–90.
12. Kevin Tanzillo, "House Call: Telemed Provides Bedside Service," *Communication News* 26 (June 1989): 47.
13. Raymond Beswick and N. L. Reinsch, Jr., "Attitudinal Responses to Voice Mail," *Journal of Business Communications* 24, no. 3 (Summer 1987): 23–35.
14. James G. Anderson, Stephen J. Jay, Harlan M. Schweer, and Marilyn M. Anderson, "Physician Utilization of Computers in Medical Practice: Policy Implications Based on a Structural Model," *Social Science and Medicine* 23, no. 3 (1986): 259–267.
15. John W. Williamson et al., "Health Science Information Management and Continuing Education of Physicians," *Annals of Internal Medicine* 110, no. 2 (January 15, 1989): 151–60.
16. David Weber, "Tuning In to Patient Channel Systems," *Healthcare Forum* (January/February 1987).
17. Linda Perry, "Guidelines Help Test Legality of Physician Computer Links," *Modern Healthcare* 19, no. 47 (November 24, 1989): 22.
18. Perry, "Guidelines," p. 22.
19. Weber, "Tuning In."
20. Weber, "Tuning In."
21. Suzanne Powills, "Hospital-Physician Link Generates $4 Million," *Hospitals* 61 (December 5, 1987).
22. Weber, "Tuning In."
23. Pamela Hanlon and E. Andrew Kaskiw, "Integrating Market Research in the Creation of Hospital/Physician Networks," *Healthcare Computing and Communications* (November 1987): 67–70.

Part IV

Case Studies

Part I

10.

Technology Acquisition and Implementation in Four Organizations

Introduction

Four case studies are presented in Part IV. The major objective in preparing these cases was to understand how managers dealt with the issues faced in acquiring and implementing technologies that could improve service quality. After a brief discussion of how the organizations were selected and the case studies prepared, some of the similar issues that were uncovered will be examined.

Selection of the Four Organizations

Only a limited number of in-depth case studies could be prepared. The objective in selecting organizations was to document a variety of management responses (for example, analyses prepared, decisions made, procedures established), rather than to make generalizations about how all organizations behave.

To assure that a variety of responses would be observed, organizations of various sizes, organizational structures, and geographic locations were selected.

The four sites were in four different regions of the United States (Northeast, Midwest, Southeast, and Southwest). Competition and economic and demographic differences have created distinctly different environments for health care organizations in these regions. Both individual hospitals and hospital systems were selected. The two individual hospitals differed greatly in size, from a 1,020-bed medical center (the Cleveland Clinic Foundation) to a 300-bed community hospital (Vassar Brothers Hospital in Poughkeepsie, New York).

The two multihospital systems were Samaritan Health Services (SHS) in Phoenix (a multihospital system that owned or operated 7 hospitals with 1,596 beds) and Inter+Net Health System (a separate corporation in the Washington, D.C., area formed by 13 not-for-profit hospitals with a total of 3,591 beds). Inter+Net Health System did not own or manage any hospitals but carried out activities considered beneficial to its members.

The response of managers could also be affected by the type of technology under consideration. A balance was struck between variety and the desire to observe managers dealing with the similar issues involved in a single type of technology. Two technologies were selected that were receiving greater attention in health care journals and conferences in 1989, hospital-to-physician computer links and physician/service referral systems.

Samaritan Health Services, Vassar Brothers Hospital, and the Cleveland Clinic were implementing a physician-to-hospital computer link. Inter+Net Health System was implementing a very different type of technology—a health information and referral system that put registered nurses in front of a personal computer and made them accessible over the phone 24 hours a day, seven days a week.

In addition to documenting how an organization went about implementing a very different type of technology, the purpose of doing the Inter+Net case was to see if some of the issues uncovered in the other three cases were important when the technology was considerably different.

Preparation of the Cases

Site visits were made to the four organizations. Managers were interviewed, documents collected for study, and the technology observed in use. Subsequent telephone and personal interviews were conducted to answer questions that arose after a draft of the case was prepared and visits were made to other organizations. Managers at each organization reviewed and commented on successive drafts of the case study.

No attempt was made to impose a conceptual framework on the cases. The cases are intended to assist managers working in information systems development, marketing, and strategic planning, as well as senior managers whose responsibilities overlap these functions. Selecting a conceptual framework from one of these areas might have limited the usefulness of the cases to this broad range of professionals. Instead, a range of topics of interest to professionals working in these areas are examined in considerable detail. The result is lengthy cases that should be useful to a wide range of professionals and demonstrate the interrelationship of marketing, strategic planning, and information systems development.

Issues Facing Managers

The discussion that follows focuses on issues facing all four organizations. The selection of issues is based on the personal judgment of the author, who believes they deserve serious consideration by anyone acquiring and implementing technology for the purpose of improving service quality. Some personal judgments by the author about the appropriateness of the decisions made by each organization are also provided. The extensive detail provided in the cases should allow readers to arrive at their own conclusions. The major issues raised by the experience of these four organizations are:

— The relationship of the technology to organizational strategy. Is it always necessary to assess a technology on the basis of short-term, measurable financial results?

— Which technology should be selected?

— How should financial performance be assessed?

— Who should be responsible and accountable for marketing the new service and assuring service quality, and how do they gain the cooperation of important internal groups?

Strategic Importance of the Technology

The experience of these four organizations suggests that the definition of a strategy, the selection of a technology, and the definition and monitoring of financial and other objectives are interrelated choices for an organization.

An organization that views the technology as a way of directly achieving specific and measurable objectives is likely to find some technologies more attractive than others. Affecting the choice of technology is the ability of the user to measure the extent to which the achievement of objectives, like increases in service volume and revenue, can be attributed to the new technology.

An organization that views the technology as only one means of pursuing a larger strategy has made another choice. Technologies that enhance services to physicians and patients may be attractive even if the direct benefits are more difficult to calculate. The challenge is to develop criteria for making the investment so that boards of trustees and other decision makers in the organization will be satisfied that ultimately the organization will benefit from the technology.

Strategy and the Use of Technology in Four Organizations

All of the organizations studied used the technology selected as a means of pursuing larger strategies. They did not view the services created with the technologies as simply a means of increasing service volume and profits. The strategies included obtaining or sustaining a high percentage of the referrals made by physicians, and obtaining a competitive advantage in negotiations with payers (for example, for a contract with a PPO).

All four organizations viewed the technology as a peripheral, rather than a core, element of the service package being offered.[1] Managers at Samaritan Health Services, the Cleveland Clinic, and Vassar Brothers Hospital believed they were providing physicians with a benefit and, therefore, helping to differentiate themselves from competing hospitals. The core elements of the service package being offered to physicians continued, however, to be services rendered to patients in the hospital.

Although Ask-A-Nurse was the core service being offered to patients by Inter+Net Health System, management justified the investment in Ask-A-Nurse in terms of the benefits to member hospitals and their physicians. In the first few years, the primary benefit was to be additional revenues to hospitals from inpatient admissions. However, Ask-A-Nurse was only the first component of a larger information system and would not be the core service that Inter+Net Health System would provide. Those core services would be the ability to collect, disseminate, and analyze the data needed to help make Inter+Net into a single system for the delivery of health care to the metropolitan area. The ultimate customer of that larger information center would be payers, who would view Inter+Net as a superior organization to do business with because of its ability to coordinate and provide access to care (as well as document the quality of the care provided).

Although the technologies created services that were peripheral to the core services provided, this does not mean they were unimportant, since peripheral services can be the primary means by which a service organization differentiates itself from competitors. The distinction between peripheral and core services is useful, however, in trying to understand the decisions made by managers, who might have acted differently if the new services were core services. For example, marketing the physician-to-hospital computer link might have been a higher priority at Samaritan Health Services, the Cleveland Clinic, and Vassar Brothers if it had been a health care service rather than a means of communicating about those services.

Did the Technology Fit the Strategy Selected?

An assessment of whether each organization selected appropriate strategies for achieving its goals in its particular community is beyond the scope of this study. It would require, for example, the collection of data on competitors and the attitudes and behaviors of patients, physicians, and payers. This was not attempted. What can be considered is whether the selection of a technology was appropriate given the strategy selected.

Since we do not have studies of the impact of these technologies that would allow a final judgment on even this issue, it is even more important to ask whether the organizations had in place a system for monitoring performance to allow decisions to be made on increases or decreases in investment.

Choosing a Technology

An organization has to both choose a generic type of technology and select a desired level of investment. The technologies come in basic and more complex and expensive versions, as described in Chapters 4 and 9. The generic characteristics of the technologies selected by these four organizations will first be reviewed, and then their level of investment discussed.

Technologies Selected

Computer links are only one medium for communication, and ease of communication is not the primary benefit that physicians are seeking from a hospital or other health care organization. This makes it difficult to establish a cause-and-effect relationship between the use of the link and referrals. On the other hand, peripheral services offered to a physician may affect behavior, especially where core services offered by two health care organizations are considered equivalent.

The development of a computer link was consistent with the strategies of the Cleveland Clinic, Samaritan Health Services, and Vassar Brothers Hospital: to develop a competitive advantage by offering physicians enhanced services that cumulatively might affect behavior. The position of Cleveland Clinic CompreLink as one service in the CompreCare program for referring physicians is the clearest example. Samaritan Health Services and Vassar Brothers, however, also had a range of benefits for physicians that included a computer link.

The fit between Inter+Net's strategy and the selection of Ask-A-Nurse is more difficult to assess because Ask-A-Nurse was relevant to several strategies. A short-range strategy of Inter+Net's management was to increase the visibility of Inter+Net and accustom its members to working together. As a way of generating visibility, as well as additional admissions that would reward voluntary cooperation, the Ask-A-Nurse product had significant potential.

The existence of substantial numbers of people in major metropolitan areas without a continuing relationship to a physician, and the interest in receiving information and assistance demonstrated by the large volume of calls received by other sites, suggested the potential for this type of technology to result in a significant volume of patients being channeled to a particular group of providers. A final judgment on this issue cannot be made, but it is possible that the costs of this technology could be justified solely on the basis of increases in service volume.

Ask-A-Nurse seems less relevant to a strategy of attracting payers. The channeling of patients to appropriate sources of care, communication of benefits information, and other services that Inter+Net Health System managers feel payers want could be provided by trained service personnel who were not nurses.

If the Ask-A-Nurse system is seen as a way of funding the first step in the development of such an information center and developing expertise in telecommunications, it appears more relevant. An information center for payers and insurance beneficiaries would have to be paid for by revenues received from payers and would require an initial investment by Inter+Net's members until contracts were signed. It might then become an important peripheral element in the service package being offered. Only time would tell if this particular service actually affected negotiations with payers.

The Ask-A-Nurse service, therefore, became a way of establishing a telecommunications capability that paid for itself but which could be converted to what a strategy toward payers required. Inter+Net Health System managers are, however, faced with the challenge of changing payer attitudes and beliefs about what the Ask-A-Nurse system does and convincing them that it can be turned into something of value for them. On the other hand, they will be able to point to thousands of consumer inquiries handled and, hopefully, a positive image among consumers.

Level of Investment

The decision on how much to invest was closely related to the choice of technology. A technology like the Ask-A-Nurse system required a much higher level of investment than a basic computer link. By choosing a computer link, an organization obtained greater flexibility in how much and when to invest funds.

The three organizations that developed a computer link used this flexibility. Each developed a pilot to test the technology and evaluate physician acceptance and satisfaction.

There were other ways to affect the investment required. Samaritan Health Services developed its own software using in-house programmers.

Vassar Brothers bought a basic package from a vendor and then extensively modified it. The Cleveland Clinic became an "alpha," or developmental, site for a vendor. None of the three signed a contract with an existing vendor for an existing system with state-of-the-art capabilities—the most expensive strategy.

Samaritan Health Services, Cleveland Clinic, and Vassar Brothers managers, therefore, solved the problem of how to convince decision makers like the board of trustees to invest in a system whose direct payoff was difficult to forecast by proceeding cautiously through a pilot phase. Samaritan Health Services and Vassar Brothers also limited investment by relying on in-house resources. The Cleveland Clinic balanced the risks of investment against the desire to obtain an innovative, clinically oriented system and settled on a joint venture with a vendor.

Managers in each organization also mentioned specific reasons for the level of investment selected. Samaritan Health Services saw itself as leveraging its existing information resources to provide a valuable service at a relatively low cost. The value obtained from its sunk costs in information systems would be increased.

Since physicians who were not members of the Cleveland Clinic staff could not treat patients there, they had no need for billing data from the Cleveland Clinic. Cleveland Clinic managers felt a system that focused on the transmission of clinical data was needed. This made the system from Integrated Medical Systems (IMS) attractive.

Vassar Brothers Hospital wanted to counteract a reputation for being less able to provide fast service because of lower staffing levels. The clients were physicians and their office staffs. The computer link could be viewed as a substitute for higher investment in personnel to answer telephones and respond to inquiries.

Inter+Net Health System's management faced a very different situation, however. Inter+Net had no funds of its own to invest. It could provide a modest service to its members for a modest investment, but it would still have to secure funds from its members.

The alternative was to do something that would make Inter+Net more visible and offer something unique, not available from its members and other providers. The Ask-A-Nurse system required a higher investment ($1.4 million was spent in 1988, and $1.5 million was budgeted for 1989) but provided a unique service. An exclusive market-area license for the Ask-A-Nurse system was available but could be purchased by another organization. The ability to document from experiences in other areas that Ask-A-Nurse could increase patient volume and profits also helped in making the decision to recommend this level of investment.

Was the level of investment of each organization appropriate? The technology selected by Inter+Net required a high level of investment to purchase an exclusive franchise and follow the service model that had proved successful elsewhere, a 24-hour-a-day, seven-day-a-week service staffed by nurses. The high call volume that had been generated elsewhere suggested that a high level of investment in staff was needed to avoid negative reactions if Inter+Net failed to deliver on its promise of access to a nurse. The multimillion dollar investment was necessary to achieve the benefits of operating such a service in a large metropolitan area.

Both SHS and Cleveland Clinic could have developed computer links that cost more than $1 million by adopting a strategy of providing physicians with a full range of free software (including practice management) and hardware, following the model of Borgess Medical Center.[2] SHS had seen St. Joseph's Hospital and Medical Center in Phoenix not succeed after investing what they believed was $4 million. It is not surprising, therefore, that SHS managers wanted to move more slowly, first defining user needs and then developing the internal capability to serve physicians.

The Cleveland Clinic wanted to use a clinically oriented system that was not yet developed. Because the technology was new, the Cleveland Clinic was correct in conducting a pilot study first. The slow growth of the link when only a modest physician payment was required also suggests that offering a free system would not have been appropriate. The Cleveland Clinic might have spent a great deal of money on a system that was accepted because it was free, and then not used or highly valued. In order to sell this service, Cleveland Clinic staff had to become oriented to the needs of physicians and their staffs.

The level of investment by Vassar Brothers is the hardest to assess. Vassar Brothers had the capability of supporting a larger system and a competitor who appeared capable and interested in moving in this direction. On the other hand, Vassar Brothers believed that its financial situation did not allow a larger investment. Since the link itself would not generate revenue, the low level of investment during a period of fiscal stress seems justified. The question is when, and if, that investment will have to be increased to effectively compete. A link with an expanded array of services could be an important element in an enhanced package of services to physicians that retains their loyalty.

Should They Have Chosen Another Technology?

Another way of considering the issue of the appropriateness of a technology to an organization's strategy is to consider whether another choice would have been as appropriate. This discussion will be limited to whether Inter+Net Health System would have been better off developing a computer link, and the other three organizations an Ask-A-Nurse system.

An Ask-A-Nurse system would not have been an appropriate investment for the Cleveland Clinic since its primary mission is to provide specialized services on referral from physicians. A system intended to be the
first contact with a patient was therefore not appropriate. A study showed that
the Cleveland Clinic received an average of $7,000 for services provided to a
patient referred by a physician, and $2,000 for patients who referred them-
selves. An Ask-A-Nurse system was not necessary to provide physicians in
the region with referrals to Cleveland Clinic physicians. This could be done
over the link.

The smaller size of the Poughkeepsie area and the limited ability of
Vassar Brothers Hospital to provide services to a dispersed rural population
through its own network of physicians would make the Ask-A-Nurse less
desirable. If Vassar Brothers advertised only in the immediate Poughkeepsie
area, it might not get a sufficient volume of calls to offset the expense. If it
advertised the service to a wide geographic area, Vassar Brothers would not
be able to meet the demand for services with its own physicians and one
hospital. Referrals would have to be made to nonaffiliated physicians and
other hospitals, with no benefit to Vassar Brothers. Alternatives would be the
development of a consortium of hospitals or a contract with an existing Ask-
A-Nurse site (see the Port Huron example in the Inter+Net case in Chapter
14).

The size of the Phoenix market and the number of facilities operated by
Samaritan Health Services could make an Ask-A-Nurse system an attractive
investment. However, this choice would not allow Samaritan Health Services
to leverage or multiply the value of its existing investment in its computer
system and data bases on patients and physicians, as with the computer link.
Of the three organizations that developed computer links, Samaritan Health
Services should be most interested in considering an Ask-A-Nurse system
because of its potential to direct patients to SHS hospitals, and to provide
services to employers, HMOs, and other third-party payers.

For Inter+Net Health System, a computer link to its hospitals and their
physicians would be a less desirable investment. Inter+Net would have to
link to a number of mainframes and minicomputers, some of which are
almost certainly incompatible. A link to physicians might also yield limited
value, since Inter+Net itself does not have the medical and billing data that
physicians need, nor does it directly provide care to the physician's patients.
Only physicians with multiple medical staff appointments and a significant
volume of patients in more than one Inter+Net Health System hospital would
find the use of a central switching station for messages to individual hospitals
attractive. Other physicians would primarily want to receive and send information from the hospitals where they treated most of their patients, since
these hospitals would have the information on services and the condition of
their patients.

Financial Objectives and Performance

As noted earlier, the definition of a strategy, the selection of a technology, and the definition and monitoring of financial and other objectives are interrelated choices for an organization. To a certain extent, the selection of a technology determined the extent to which financial objectives could be defined and their attainment measured. Some technologies have effects that are difficult to isolate and measure, while others produce results that can be. The extent to which these organizations defined financial objectives and attempted to measure their attainment is first discussed, and then some possible explanations for their actions are explored.

Defining and Measuring Financial Performance

The managers of these organizations did not take some actions that would be expected if they were interested in investing in these technologies primarily because of their ability to directly achieve higher service volumes or profits.

Assessments of impact

During the period covered by the case studies, only the Cleveland Clinic actually completed a study to determine the impact of a technology on service volume. The study showed an increase of four referrals per site (for outpatient or inpatient services) over a six-month period. This study was not repeated during the period covered by the case, although the Cleveland Clinic planned to make it routine. Samaritan Health Services and Inter+Net Health System also had plans for routine assessment.

Two of the four sites (which included 25 of the 29 physicians linked) selected by Vassar Brothers for the pilot were the offices of physicians who admitted all of their inpatients to Vassar Brothers. Vassar Brothers made no attempt to determine whether there were additional admissions from the other sites, a solo practice and a three-person group.

Financial forecasts

Samaritan Health Services and Inter+Net Health System were the only two organizations that developed financial plans that included forecasts of both revenues and expenses. The SHS financial forecast used alternative assumptions about the number of incremental admissions per installation (i.e., a physician's office). SHS estimated, for example, that if half of the installations had existing hardware and the other half required that SHS provide hardware (with the physician paying for it over a five-year period), and each installation generated two more admissions per year, the link would be profitable in the second year of operation.

A reason for favoring an estimate of zero, two, or four incremental admissions per installation was not presented and would be very difficult to defend in any case. It was important, however, for Samaritan Health Services to do this analysis to clarify for senior management the impact of no incremental admissions vs. some impact. Senior managers could then look at the worst-case scenario—no additional admissions—and judge whether other unquantified benefits would still make the investment worthwhile. One of the benefits was an increase in the utilization of some outpatient services. Another was the possibility of earlier discharge of patients if diagnostic test results were provided on a timely basis.

The financial plan for Inter+Net's Ask-A-Nurse system included a financial forecast that used assumptions derived by examining the experience of other Ask-A-Nurse sites around the United States. Conservative assumptions were selected, and the financial implications calculated. A sensitivity analysis was then performed of two assumptions, the percent of hospital admissions that were actually due to the Ask-A-Nurse system (those that the hospital would not have gotten anyway) and the marginal cost of treating patients. The analysis showed that the Ask-A-Nurse system was financially unattractive only if marginal hospital revenue was less than 35 percent (i.e., more than 65 percent of the revenues would have been received anyway) and marginal hospital cost was more than 40 percent of marginal revenue.

Inter+Net Health System, therefore, engaged in a more sophisticated analysis of the extent to which its investment was dependent on some critical assumptions underlying the use of both computer links and referrals systems to increase service volume—that the events attributed to the technology would have happened anyway and that hospitals would not incur large marginal costs in meeting the increased demand. Hospitals with significant unused capacity would be less concerned than Inter+Net Health System with the latter issue, especially in the case of inpatient care, where the ratio of fixed to variable costs is higher.

Issues and Problems

Measuring the actual use of services

Defining and measuring financial performance can be difficult because of the characteristics of a specific technology. One such characteristic of both computer links and service referral systems is that the data stored by the technology itself is not the definitive source of information on whether a service was used. A patient may be referred to a physician by the Ask-A-Nurse nurse, but fail to make an appointment. The nurse may make the appointment, but the patient may not keep it. The only way to find out what actually happened is to contact the physician or other provider, or examine the bill for services. Inter+Net Health System intended to do this by reconciling (matching) hospital bills from its 13 hospitals with data on callers stored in the Ask-A-Nurse computer.

Determining the impact of a computer link would also require such a reconciliation. Services requested using the link could be compared to services actually used if the computer stored the name and other characteristics of a patient to allow a match to hospital records. None of the three organizations developing a computer link planned to do such a reconciliation. The SHS and Vassar Brothers systems did not allow a physician to order a service. The Cleveland Clinic system allowed a request for a referral to be entered, but such a request could also be made through a general message function. There was, therefore, no way to determine the total number of services requested without examining each message, a tedious process that the Cleveland Clinic did not plan to go through.

One clear improvement in measurement for referral systems would be to reconcile the data stored by the system to physicians' office records or bills. This would require either that physician office staff compare records (which they may not wish, or have the time, to do) or that physicians provide their bills (which they may not want to do to protect the confidentiality of their business records).

Did the technology alter behavior?

Another dilemma is how to determine if the technology resulted in a referral, that is, whether it occurred only because the technology was used. Since patients and physicians can communicate with each other and with hospitals over the telephone, in person, and in writing, it is difficult to say whether a computer link or referral system was responsible for a service being delivered. The volume of calls or referrals on the system itself is not an accurate measure of additional service volume.

The problem is greater for technologies like a physician-to-hospital link, where current physicians are being served, than for referral systems, where patients without a regular physician they are satisfied with are the primary clients. The Ask-A-Nurse system, which provides information as well as a referral, falls somewhere in between. Patients currently using Inter+Net physicians may also be calling just for information. In these cases, the ultimate effect may be higher patient satisfaction, but no increase in service volume.

Hospitals and other health care organizations considering an investment in technology that are concerned with obtaining a higher volume of new services should first consider the physician and service referral technology because it is easier to estimate the actual increase in service use that is due to the technology. The degree to which a hospital-to-physician computer link will increase the loyalty of existing physicians and help sustain an existing market share is not known at this time.

Effect of physician selection on financial performance

The most dramatic impact would occur if physicians who had split admissions or not used the hospital changed their behavior. On the other hand, a hospital may feel that loyal physicians have to be included first to prevent dissatisfaction and, perhaps, a loss of referrals. Loyal physicians, however, provide little incremental revenue. Managers at Vassar Brothers decided not to try to measure increases in admissions because 25 of the 29 physicians in the pilot admitted all of their patients to Vassar Brothers.

The need to serve loyal physicians and those who split admissions results in several measurement and assessment problems. The inclusion of loyalists incurs costs, but increased revenues are unlikely to result. On the other hand, a loss of revenues when loyal physicians use competing hospitals may be averted by improving the service package offered. The financial impact of a link may be understated when we only look for new revenues. There is no way to estimate the loss of admissions from loyal physicians that would have occurred if the computer link had not been established. The reasons for a physician changing behavior are difficult to determine. Even an interview does not necessarily provide a valid explanation of why a change was made. What a physician reports as the cause of shifting referrals may not have been what produced the change in behavior.

Both the Cleveland Clinic and Samaritan Health Services chose a mix of physicians, including those who provided a large share of their referrals to the organization and those who managers felt could provide significantly more. Although the Cleveland Clinic offers any new CompreCare physician the opportunity to use CompreLink, it targets certain physicians who they believe could provide additional referrals. Physician service representatives actively promote CompreLink to these physicians. Samaritan Health Services has also developed a prioritization process for its marketing efforts.

Determining the financial impact of physician and service referral systems poses fewer problems than determining the impact of a computer link. It is easier to assume that a patient who calls looking for a physician would not have been admitted to a specific hospital unless the patient was referred to a physician on the medical staff. Attributing referrals to a computer link asks us to estimate the significance of one medium for communication in the decision-making process of a physician.

Although the four organizations studied could invest additional resources in reconciling patients and callers, as well as tracking the number of referrals, only sophisticated surveys and observational research concerning physician behavior are likely to yield evidence of the effect of how physicians communicate on where and what they order. Robert Ludke and Gary Levitz describe the results of such a study and provide other sources of information on this type of research.[3]

Decisions Made and Future Directions

None of the four organizations moved through all of the steps involved in defining and measuring financial performance: the definition of performance measures, forecasting of performance, and performance measurement. Inter-+Net and Samaritan Health Services had completed the first two. At the time the cases were written, both organizations were in the early stages of implementation and had plans to complete the last step. It is not possible to assess whether each organization could have proceeded more quickly to measure actual performance.

Vassar Brothers Hospital was completing a pilot test, and managers had begun to discuss issues that needed to be resolved before financial performance measures could be established. These included whether physicians would be given computer systems and which physicians—loyalists or splitters—would be favored. Vassar Brothers clearly needed to move ahead in the process of financial planning in order to justify a larger investment to its board. Selecting primarily physicians for the pilot who admitted all of their patients to Vassar Brothers was a political choice whose appropriateness cannot be evaluated. Vassar Brothers might have suffered a loss of patient volume if current physicians who were unhappy (about not receiving the equipment or services in general) had chosen to admit their patients elsewhere, while those physicians who split admission did not increase their volume sufficiently to make up the loss.

The Cleveland Clinic was the only organization that had actually conducted a study of changes in referral patterns. Managers had plans to monitor changes in the number of referrals by site each quarter. Financial performance was to be measured by multiplying the number of both inpatient and outpatient referrals (totaled together) by the average revenue received from all physicians (including those not on CompreLink). This would not indicate the net revenue received from referrals by CompreLink physicians. This method was considerably easier to use and required less data than directly measuring gross and net revenue by CompreLink physicians. It is not possible to determine from the information collected for the case how difficult a physician-specific measurement of net revenue would have been, but such a system would be clearly superior.

The Cleveland Clinic also faced the problem of determining the volume of referrals that could be attributed to the use of CompreLink. Trends in the number of referrals could only suggest, rather than demonstrate, that CompreLink was changing physician behavior. Studies of changes in physician attitudes and behavior that would supplement the measurement of trends in referrals were needed. Physician service representatives could be used for such studies since they visited each physician office quarterly.

Responsibility and Accountability for Marketing and Service Quality

Growth and service excellence can be sustained partly by developing the appropriate organizational structure (i.e., defining who is responsible and accountable), but to a greater extent depends on getting individuals and groups in the organization to accept growth and service quality as a personal goal. The discussion that follows describes the organizational structure selected to manage the service created by the new technology, but focuses on the issue of how each organization dealt with important internal groups.

Organization and Internal Marketing

In the cases of the Cleveland Clinic and Samaritan Health Services, an existing unit of the organization was given the lead role in developing the service but had to negotiate to obtain the cooperation and compliance of other units of the organization that were either peers or had superior prestige and authority. The task, as might be expected, was to market the system internally to achieve the compliance that they did not have the authority to secure.

In the case of the Cleveland Clinic, the unit was the Division of Physician Liaison and Alumni Affairs. The division managers in charge of the CompreLink program had to obtain the commitment of several internal groups.

The provision of "overreads" (i.e., an interpretation of test data sent over the link) raised problems for Cleveland Clinic managers since it required that Cleveland Clinic physicians agree to provide this service in a timely manner. They were able to obtain the agreement of pulmonary specialists to do this, but not cardiologists. They did not seek or obtain promises concerning how quickly physicians would provide an overread, although timely service was a critical element for success.

To get pulmonary specialists to provide overreads of pulmonary function tests, they had to take a series of steps to assure them that the data received would be accurate. A respiratory therapist at the Cleveland Clinic was hired by the vendor to be their field representative. This individual trained the office staff who would perform the test at a two-day session at the

Cleveland Clinic and was present when the first one was performed at a physician's office.

One of the major potential benefits of CompreLink for physicians was the timely transmission of information on what occurred to their patients at the Cleveland Clinic so that the physician appeared knowledgeable and could plan appropriate follow-up treatment. This required the multiple departments that patients (especially inpatients) came into contact with to compile and transmit patient information quickly. To speed up the process, the Cleveland Clinic intended to hire a registered nurse to compile the information and see that it was transmitted over CompreLink immediately.

Senior managers at Samaritan Health Services decided to give responsibility for the Pulse system (a physician-to-hospital computer link) to the Information Services Department. However, to assure that the marketing of the Pulse system was coordinated with other physician service activities, the marketing director of each SHS hospital was asked to market Pulse by making the initial contact with physicians. Pulse staff would then install the system, train staff, and evaluate user satisfaction. Although this seemed logical, it left Pulse staff with an internal marketing problem. They had to make sure that marketing staff were making Pulse a priority.

A second issue was that selling the Pulse system to many physicians involved immediately explaining the costs and convincing the physician's staff that it could help them do their jobs. Marketing directors lacked the technical expertise to determine the hardware requirements and cost for each physician, and to show physician office staff how the system would help them do their jobs. Samaritan Health Services had started out seeing the physician as the customer, but the staff may have a more important role once the physician thinks the cost is acceptable.

The SHS managers felt that this division of responsibility slowed the growth of the network. The issue was resolved when Information Services took over the marketing of Pulse, partly because of the departure of marketing staff at SHS hospitals. Information Services staff selected physicians from prioritized lists prepared by each hospital and contacted the administrator in charge of physician relations prior to calling a physician. Information Services staff then proceeded to make the presentation directly.

The issue facing organizations that want to use such intermediaries to promote computer-based services is how to make those intermediaries give this activity a high priority and how to assure that they can answer questions about cost and performance. A physician-technician team is one possible answer, but this will require commitment from physicians to a team effort. This option is most feasible in organizations where physicians have a sense of ownership (through financial investment or direct control as in the Cleveland Clinic) or where salaried physician executives are used.

Inter+Net Health System created a separate organization to develop Ask-A-Nurse that included its own manager, nurse supervisors, technical services manager, and marketing director. Although Inter+Net Health System developed the organization, Ask-A-Nurse was designed to be spun off as a separate corporation. Inter+Net did not, therefore, have to coordinate the efforts of staff from multiple hospitals working on the Ask-A-Nurse project, but they still had to take their commitment into consideration. Inter+Net relied on its member hospitals and their physicians to deliver high-quality services.

Inter+Net managers perceived that hospital marketing directors viewed Inter+Net as competing with their own programs for resources, even though the benefits would accrue to their hospitals. One group of hospitals in the Inter+Net system was spending approximately $2 million per year on their own physician referral system. A major question was whether, and how, to integrate the efforts of its own members and their staffs into what Inter+Net was doing. Inter+Net decided not to integrate other physician referral systems, but to create a separate system with a considerably different approach. None of the other systems operating in Inter+Net member hospitals used a nurse to provide information and assessments. By choosing a considerably different product, Inter+Net sought to reduce any sense of competition and create a complementary and not entirely competitive service.

The potential for tension remained, however, since funds provided by members could be defined as marketing funds not allocated to a hospital's own marketing department. Since Ask-A-Nurse does not directly generate revenues, Inter+Net Health System must return each year to its member hospitals and ask for funds for the existing Ask-A-Nurse system and any improvements and additions.

Vassar Brothers Hospital also assigned responsibility for its computer link to the Information Systems Department. The director of that department reported to the vice-president of Professional/Support Services. For this project, the vice-president of Corporate Development was actively involved. Vassar Brothers Hospital, with 300 beds, was a much smaller organization. There was daily contact among senior managers. As a single hospital, there was no question of the benefits of the link accruing to a larger corporate entity rather than to an individual hospital.

The major issue facing Vassar was how to make the transition from viewing the link system as an Information Systems Department activity to a routine physician service. The director of Information Systems had begun to see that maintenance and growth of this system as it stabilized did not require the skills of his staff. Physician staff training and support, rather than programming skills, were needed. Vassar Brothers managers were left with the issue of how to define and compensate a new type of employee, one who had primarily marketing and training functions but who could deal with some of the technical issues involved in a computer-based system.

At Samaritan Health Services, the question was where among the existing units to assign responsibility. In a small organization like Vassar, the issue was how to define and compensate an individual who would work with several senior managers and meet several needs at the same time.

Decisions Made and Future Directions

Both SHS and Vassar Brothers chose to give their information services/ systems departments the responsibility for developing the new service created. Since they both chose to develop or customize a link without major assistance from a vendor, this was appropriate. The technical problems involved in developing the system were likely to require that the information systems departments have the major responsibility. This decision needs to be reconsidered as the system matures and the technical elements of the link are less of a concern. The link is a promise of service, and what physicians and their office staffs will be looking for is current and accurate patient information.

The experience of the Cleveland Clinic suggests that service excellence will require the ability to assemble and transmit clinical information in response to inquiries, and the clinical departments will play a major role. All four organizations have already begun to address this issue by giving management positions to staff with clinical training and experience. A major question for SHS is whether they need to move further to create a sense of ownership among clinicians. This might be accomplished by the creation of a unit to operate Pulse in which they have more direct involvement. The physician liaison division at the Cleveland Clinic is one model.

Vassar Brothers faces the same problem and may respond by the development of an interdepartmental unit reporting to both Hospital Operations and Corporate Development. Physician involvement in the management of such a unit should be considered.

Inter+Net has appropriately chosen to establish a separate unit and to spin it off. It is difficult to imagine how Ask-A-Nurse could have been quickly established as a joint venture of 13 hospitals with the division of responsibility among members.

The Cleveland Clinic decision to make the Division of Physician Liaison and Alumni Affairs responsible for the computer link seems both appropriate and a model for how this type of technology could be implemented. The emphasis is on service, and senior physicians are involved. Reliance on the vendor is very high, however, and the Cleveland Clinic needs to consider how internal information systems professionals or outside consultants might be brought into the decision-making process to advise on future directions. The Cleveland Clinic planned to hire a staff member with technical skills for this purpose. Technical considerations should not, however, be allowed to dominate decision making and reduce the emphasis on service.

Internal marketing, that is, marketing to groups and individuals within the organization, is clearly the most important challenge facing all four organizations. In the final section of this chapter, the concept of exchange will be discussed to provide some advice to other organizations interested in implementing this type of technology.

Managers at the Cleveland Clinic, SHS, and Vassar Brothers all had to make decisions about how much effort to devote to internal marketing as opposed to dealing with the technical problems of establishing a computer link. It is impossible to say how much in the way of staff and other resources should have been reallocated to internal marketing efforts like personal communications and training. Technical problems are immediate, obvious to everyone, and can be fixed. Internal marketing problems create no emergencies, and their signs and solutions are often not obvious. As each organization leaves the period when technical problems demand resolution, they need to devote more resources to educating important internal groups and developing ways to obtain their cooperation and commitment, a subject that will be discussed later.

Inter+Net's internal marketing problems will be less significant if the financial payoff to member hospitals is as large as expected. Inter+Net managers have made some shrewd choices. They selected a noncompeting service with a potentially large payoff that most of their individual members could not afford to start, and benefit from, on their own. The major challenges will come in the next stage of development, when Inter+Net tries to provide services like claims processing that require the transfer of functions from the individual hospital and physician to Inter+Net. Inter+Net will face the challenge of obtaining a high level of cooperation and commitment to its managers' vision of how a regional health care system should operate. The concept of exchange discussed later will be critically important. The Inter+Net board and other influential groups will also have to be educated and involved in the decision-making process.

Implications for Other Organizations

The Relationship of Strategy to Technology Selected

Hospitals that are interested in stand-alone services with a separate, measurable financial impact should, therefore, look more closely at physician/service referral systems, both basic systems and systems like Ask-A-Nurse. As part of a larger strategy of improving communications with physicians and creating organized systems of care, the hospital-to-physician computer link deserves serious attention, although the specific benefits are likely to be harder to measure.

The major error that an organization could make is selecting a technology that is not well suited to the desired objective. If immediate financial results are needed, for example, the hospital-to-physician computer link would not be the best choice, although it may yield a significant competitive advantage for a hospital pursuing a strategy of enhancing services to physicians to obtain and sustain their loyalty.

Organizations that follow the example of these four organizations and view the technologies as only one way of pursuing a strategy will be able to select technologies that may have long-run benefits, although their short-term, identifiable results may be limited. Those who establish stand-alone services with clearly defined financial objectives may more easily justify the investment to cost-conscious boards of trustees and CEOs. The internal staff, financial and other resources available, and the intensity of competition will have a major effect on which course a health care organization can pursue.

The amount that needs to be invested varies with the type of technology selected and the desired results. The investment required for a hospital-to-physician computer link can vary tremendously, but so can the results. Other technologies, like the Ask-A-Nurse system, have what economists call high entry costs, that is, there is a large investment required to yield significant results. Health care organizations need to examine the experience of other organizations and use it to estimate the level of investment that may be required to yield results in the desired range.

Other decisions can be affected by the decision to view the technology as primarily supporting a larger strategy (for example, retention of market share by increasing physician satisfaction, providing services to employers and third-party payers to assist in contract negotiation). Since some strategies are considered long-range, the period that decision makers will wait before seeing significant results can be longer. This can affect decisions on when, and by how much, to increase investment in a technology, and the length of time before phasing out a service that is not producing results. On the other hand, organizations looking for significant short-term results need to be prepared to commit the funds necessary for quick, effective implementation of the new service.

Defining and Measuring Financial Performance

Defining and measuring financial performance requires both the collection/acquisition of information on what services were provided and some determination of what actually affected behavior. The collection/acquisition of information will require cooperation by other groups inside and outside of the organization, as well as computer and other resources.

Organizations that begin a service with the intention of providing short-term financial results need to budget and prepare for studies of what the results actually were, and to realize that such studies are harder for some technologies than others. Technologies like physician-to-hospital computer links can be assessed only if research is conducted, or assumptions are made, about what caused physicians and patients to use a service.

Health care organizations that use the technology to better serve loyal physicians and patients should also realize that the impact of doing so is even harder to measure since it requires making assumptions about what people might have done if a new service was not offered.

Marketing and Assuring Service Quality

In regard to marketing and assuring service quality, the experiences of these organizations suggest several issues. First, it is clear that internal marketing of the service created by a technology is critically important. If the staff and professionals involved do not understand the new service and its objectives, they cannot provide excellent service. In larger complex organizations like the Cleveland Clinic, internal marketing will require formal communication through print and other media as well as personal contacts. Where physician compliance and participation are needed, peer communication is especially important. In smaller organizations like Vassar Brothers, informal communication may suffice to win the approval and support of senior managers, but a strategy for communicating with important internal groups will still be needed.[4]

The concept of exchange has been applied by Stephen Shortell[5] to physician referral behavior, and by Philip Kotler and Roberta Clarke[6] to the question of how a health care organization obtains the resources it desires from both internal and external groups. The concept is relevant here to the internal marketing of a new service created by a technology. Managers who need the active support of other members of the organization need to consider what it is exchanging with them. If nothing of value is being exchanged, it will be very difficult to obtain the commitment of important groups and individuals.

For example, senior managers may give their support to a new service in return for support of their own projects. It is important to consider consciously what is being exchanged with groups at all levels of the organization. What are loyal physicians getting from a computer link provided free of charge to physicians who now split their admissions? If the answer is nothing, then why should they support this use of the hospital's funds? What is a marketing director (who is being evaluated on short-term results) getting from having funds allocated to the Information Services department for a service like a computer link that offers a long-range, but not a short-range, potential to boost service volume?

There can be no general answer to the question of what needs to be exchanged with various groups in return for their active support of a new service. Marketing directors can be provided with the opportunity to promote other services using the new technology (for example, using a computer link to transmit information quickly on final arrangements for a health fair, or to enroll patients in health promotion programs). Loyal physicians can be provided access to the new technology even though revenues will not increase.

The marketing of a new service created by a technology, as well as assuring consistently high service quality, requires a consideration of what is being exchanged with individuals and groups at various levels of the organization. If the answer is nothing, their support cannot be expected.

The Cases that Follow

After reading the earlier parts of this book and the cases that follow, the reader should be able to prepare at least a preliminary list of the issues and topics that their own organization will have to focus on as the acquisition and implementation of a technology is considered.

The reason for the considerable length of each of the cases is to make them interesting and informative for several audiences: senior managers responsible for overall management and strategy, marketing professionals, and information systems professionals. It is hoped that the information provided will be helpful to all three groups and will suggest the importance of collaboration and coordination of their skills and knowledge.

Notes

1. See the discussion of these concepts in Chapter 2 and in Richard Normann, *Service Management: Strategy and Leadership in Service Businesses* (Chichester, England: John Wiley & Sons, 1984).
2. David Weber, "Tuning In to Patient Channel Systems," *Healthcare Forum* (January/ February 1987).
3. Robert L. Ludke and Gary S. Levitz, "Referring Physicians: The Forgotten Market," *Health Care Management Review* (Fall 1983): 13–22.
4. Wendy Leebov, *Service Excellence: The Customer Relations Strategy for Health Care* (Chicago: American Hospital Association 1988), pp. 145–84.
5. Stephen M. Shortell, "Determinants of Physician Referral Rates: An Exchange Theory Approach," *Medical Care* 12, no. 1 (January 1974): 13–31.
6. Philip Kotler and Roberta N. Clarke, *Marketing for Health Care Organizations* (Englewood Cliffs, New Jersey: Prentice-Hall, 1987), pp. 45–52.

11.

The Cleveland Clinic Foundation's Development of a Hospital-to-Physician Computer Link

Introduction

The Cleveland Clinic Foundation is located in Cleveland, Ohio. It provided 700,000 outpatient visits and 32,000 admissions in 1988 in its outpatient facilities and a 1,020-bed hospital, which had an average occupancy of 75 percent.

All of the 600 physicians and research scientists on the staff of this not-for-profit group practice are paid salaries, and each has a vote in selecting the Board of Governors (the physician governing body of the Cleveland Clinic). Staff physicians do not practice outside of the hospital, nor can physicians not on staff treat their patients in the Cleveland Clinic's facilities.

Strategic planning and marketing are carried out by the approximately 90 staff in the Division of Public Affairs and Corporate Development. The division is active in a broad range of other activities, including government

This case was prepared by Roger Kropf, Ph.D., for publication and use in classroom discussion, rather than to illustrate either effective or ineffective handling of an administrative situation. The author wishes to thank the following Cleveland Clinic Foundation managers for their generous support in the preparation of this case: Judith A. Lester, Director of Physician Liaison and Alumni Affairs; Cynthia A. Rose, Medical Service Manager; and Frank J. Weaver, Chairman of the Division of Public Affairs and Corporate Development. Thanks also to the Cleveland Clinic staff and affiliated physicians who provided important information and insights for the development of this case.

affairs, fund development, consumer affairs (ombudsman, patient welcome program, health promotion), marketing, market research and strategic planning, communications, and physician liaison and alumni affairs. The division has developed a strong alumni association of former staff, who number over 4,000 physicians, most of whom do not practice in the local area.

In October 1987, the Cleveland Clinic began a pilot project that linked 22 physicians to the hospital by a computer link. This pilot, called Cleveland Clinic CompreLink, was part of a larger program, called Cleveland Clinic CompreCare, whose objective was to strengthen the relationships between the Cleveland Clinic and the physicians who referred patients to it. After the end of the pilot in March 1988, the Board of Governors approved the full implementation of CompreLink.

This case describes the environment faced by Cleveland Clinic managers and the strategy for increasing physician referrals they developed, the process of marketing and implementing the CompreLink system, the technical procedures and functions of the system, and its status as of early 1989.

Market Area and Competitive Environment

The Cleveland Clinic considers its local market to be the 21 counties of northeastern Ohio. It also serves a regional market that it defines as the remaining counties in Ohio and neighboring counties in Michigan, Indiana, Kentucky, New York, Pennsylvania, and West Virginia.

In 1988, 78.5 percent of outpatients came from the local market, 15.6 percent from the regional, 4.4 percent from the national, and 1.5 percent from the Cleveland Clinic's international market. The distribution for inpatients was 69 percent local, 22 percent regional, 7 percent national, and 2 percent international.

Management believes that its primary customers are the physicians, third-party payers, and patients of this local and regional market. The Cleveland Clinic has developed an array of programs to serve the needs of these three groups.

A factor that has increased competition is the aging population of northeastern Ohio, which has seen little growth as younger people leave (and fail to move in) because of the declining number of jobs in basic manufacturing industries.

Competitors

The Cleveland Clinic believes it has two types of competitors. The first group includes major academic teaching centers such as the Henry Ford Hospital in Detroit, the University of Michigan Hospitals, and the Mayo Clinic. The

Cleveland Clinic competes with these hospitals for local, regional, national, and international referrals.

The Cleveland Clinic followed the Mayo Clinic into Florida in 1987, opening its first major satellite—Cleveland Clinic Florida—in Fort Lauderdale, 325 miles south of Mayo's satellite in Jacksonville. Since 1985, the Cleveland Clinic has also developed affiliation agreements with clinics and medical institutes in Brazil, Turkey, West Germany, and England in an attempt to expand its international referrals.

The second group of competitors includes community hospitals that have upgraded their ability to provide specialized services. These community hospitals have been able to do this because of the arrival of subspecialist physicians graduating from medical schools and residency programs, including physicians trained by the Cleveland Clinic itself. Management believes that a specialized facility such as the Cleveland Clinic, linked to a large base of community physicians, can effectively compete with community hospitals seeking to establish positions as secondary and tertiary facilities.

They believe community hospitals face several disadvantages in competing with academic medical centers such as the Cleveland Clinic. First, they cannot afford to continually acquire the latest technology and other resources. Second, they cannot perform enough procedures and treat enough patients to achieve the best outcomes when compared to the larger centers. The result will be a lower quality of care that will be recognized by third-party payers and consumers. Since physicians will feel threatened when their local hospitals fail to compete effectively, they will increasingly want alliances with large medical centers.

While the Cleveland Clinic does not seek competition with community hospitals, management believes it has to be prepared to compete by developing physician-to-physician contacts. Management also believes that the Cleveland Clinic can develop collaborative and complementary roles for some community hospitals. A relationship with selected hospitals in its regional market would allow the Cleveland Clinic to demonstrate to third-party payers that it can track patients back into their local communities and assure that they receive high-quality, cost-effective care.

In 1988, a group of five hospitals from outside of the Cleveland Clinic local market asked for an affiliation agreement with the Cleveland Clinic. In response, Cleveland Clinic management developed the concept of a "hub hospital," that is, a hospital outside of the Cleveland Clinic local market area (and therefore not competing for local patients) that would channel patients to the Cleveland Clinic. Hub hospitals would be asked to assist in getting their physicians to become CompreCare affiliate physicians and to pay (or split with their physicians) the cost of joining the CompreLink program.

The five hospitals were requesting that the Cleveland Clinic provide services at their sites, something the Cleveland Clinic had never done before. As of early 1989, the Board of Governors were deliberating on what services, if any, the Cleveland Clinic might offer in these hospitals.

Employers and Third-Party Payers

Cleveland Clinic management believes that the payer should be treated as a client and customer, rather than as an adversary. Management believes that a medical center that can demonstrate high quality at a competitive price will obtain a competitive advantage in negotiating with employers and other third-party payers.

The Cleveland Clinic sought and obtained designation from the Prudential Insurance Company as an "Institute of Quality" in 1988. This designation qualifies the Cleveland Clinic to obtain exclusive contracts to provide certain services to patients enrolled in one of Prudential's managed care plans.

The Cleveland Clinic also began in 1988 to offer contracts to employers and third-party payers to provide, for a fixed price, all the hospital and professional care involved in any of 22 episodes of care. Examples are a coronary bypass with catheterization, major joint procedures, and a liver transplant. The unit price depends on the payer's volume, speed of payment, and whether the Cleveland Clinic is given an exclusive contract.

Services to Patients

The Cleveland Clinic regularly assesses patient satisfaction through telephone surveys and mail questionnaires. A "professional shopper" program is also used. The program uses trained researchers who pose as patients and report on the treatment they received. Services are also sought over the telephone and by mail, and the response evaluated.[1] The Cleveland Clinic also conducts research on the effectiveness of its efforts to promote its services to patients through various media such as direct mail and magazine articles.[2]

The Cleveland Clinic built a 400-room hotel to serve out-of-town patients and their families. Another facility with 265 beds was opened in 1988 to serve those who spend extended periods of time near the Cleveland Clinic.

The need for improvement in how services were provided was revealed by a cancelation study that examined the reasons why patients failed to keep or canceled appointments. The first hypothesis was that patients believed the Cleveland Clinic was expensive. However, problems concerning access to the Cleveland Clinic's services were cited more often.

Sometimes patients would arrive, and physicians would not be present because of other commitments. However, patients would not have been told.

Patients also complained that they were not offered choices of appointment times and dates, but were simply mailed cards that showed the date and time that had been scheduled for them. Patients also complained that they were bounced from one department and physician to another at the Cleveland Clinic. To deal with this problem, the Cleveland Clinic developed a computer-based complaint monitoring system, where complaints made by patients are entered and then followed until some action has been taken.

Physicians

There are 25,000 physicians in the region who have referred patients over time to the Cleveland Clinic. Six to seven thousand actively refer in a single year. The Cleveland Clinic needs referring physicians because it does not have the community hospital's sources of patients. It provides no primary or family care and offers no obstetrical services. It relies almost entirely on referring physicians and self-referrals by patients.

The Cleveland Clinic does provide physicals for executives through the Department of Preventive Medicine. It also opened an "Access Center" staffed by one physician and residents. Patients who call the Cleveland Clinic directly and say they are sick are referred to the Access Center for evaluation.

Referrals from physicians are, however, more desirable from a financial point of view. Referrals by physicians produce more revenue than self-referrals by patients. A study done by Cleveland Clinic staff showed that the Cleveland Clinic received an average of $7,000 for a patient referred to the Cleveland Clinic by a physician, but an average of only $2,000 for patients who referred themselves, because many patients who self-referred had minor or no problems. The referring physician, therefore, acted to triage patients and increased the efficiency with which Cleveland Clinic resources were used.

In 1983, management began to see a decline in physician referrals. It believed this decline was due not only to the growing capabilities of community hospitals, but also to the retiring of the physician population that it relied on for referrals and its replacement by physicians with little allegiance to the Cleveland Clinic. Some of them had also graduated from medical centers and teaching hospitals in the Midwest and were referring their patients to those hospitals.

Because the Cleveland Clinic wanted to reverse the trend of declining physician referrals, it conducted a study of physicians who had made referrals regularly up to 1984 and then stopped during the 1985–86 period. It surveyed a sample of those physicians to determine the reason for stopping. While some physicians had retired, a majority said that the Cleveland Clinic was not responsive to their needs or accessible to them and their patients. When asked why they used other facilities, they cited instances where those facilities called them and, in other ways, provided some personal interaction to help them keep track of their patient's care.

From this and other research, management concluded that physicians were interested in feeling more a part of the Cleveland Clinic. They wanted increased communication and a sense that they were a respected part of the Clinic's operations. The research emphasized that referrals were physician-to-physician rather than to the Cleveland Clinic itself for a specific test or procedure.

Strategy for Increasing Physician Referrals

A number of factors shaped the development of a strategy for strengthening the relationship of the Cleveland Clinic to its local and regional referring physicians. The Cleveland Clinic Foundation had been founded by a group of surgeons and had a long history of commitment to serving community physicians. Members of the Board of Governors of the Cleveland Clinic had the opportunity to hear directly from community physicians during meetings held to discuss the development of an HMO, where criticisms about access and communication were voiced. This was a critical element in moving the board to consider changes.

A major factor assisting the Cleveland Clinic in changing its physicians' attitudes and behavior toward local and regional physicians was the very real stake that Cleveland Clinic physicians had in the success of the organization. Each physician has a vote in electing the Board of Governors and does not receive salaries from other organizations, such as medical schools. This may have made it easier for the Cleveland Clinic to attempt to improve the level of services to community physicians.

Management also saw improved relations with referring physicians as essential for implementing its strategy toward hospitals and payers. Cleveland Clinic management was increasingly concerned by the potential growth in HMOs, PPOs, and other forms of managed care. It was widely believed that a larger and larger portion of the population would be locked into those ar-rangements, decreasing the number of referrals that were made to the Cleveland Clinic.

The Cleveland Clinic had to be prepared to participate in managed care plans such as HMOs or PPOs. Since the Cleveland Clinic did not provide the full spectrum of care, it would have to ally itself with a base of community physicians who could provide primary services and to whom the Cleveland Clinic could return patients following secondary and tertiary treatment.

Management envisioned three potential relationships between the Cleveland Clinic and local and regional physicians.

1. Every referring physician could become an affiliate.
2. A much smaller number would become associates by joining the Cleveland Clinic PPO.
3. An even smaller number would work as employees of the Cleveland Clinic.

The affiliate program was entitled "Cleveland Clinic CompreCare" and is described below. As of early 1989, the Cleveland Clinic had not developed a PPO or hired physicians to practice outside of the Cleveland Clinic facilities in downtown Cleveland.

Cleveland Clinic CompreCare

To recognize the importance of affiliates and provide them with some of the benefits of participation in Cleveland Clinic activities (without allowing them to practice there), the Cleveland Clinic developed a program called "Cleveland Clinic CompreCare." Any physician can join. There are no dues, but an application is required. The program had 3,100 members in April 1989.

Physicians receive the following benefits:

— preferred access to the clinic for scheduling and other communications, using a 24-hour, 7-day-a-week hotline
— access over the telephone to consulting physicians 24 hours a day, 7 days a week
— a 35 percent discount on continuing medical education (CME) courses, some of which are self-study courses
— an identification card that offers a range of benefits, including free parking at the clinic and hotel discounts when attending CME courses
— access to the clinic's placement program, which helps residents trained at the clinic to find jobs after completing their training

The major purpose of CompreCare was to significantly improve the quality of the services offered to physicians by meeting their perceived needs.

The Cleveland Clinic took a number of other steps to reduce the decline in referrals. It began producing a staff directory with photos, qualifications, and areas of specialization for all of the staff of the Cleveland Clinic and mailed this to referring physicians in its region. It also developed *Consult Magazine,* which it mails to 75,000 physicians to make them aware of services available at the Cleveland Clinic.

Development of Cleveland Clinic CompreLink

Objectives

To increase the value of its affiliate program, Cleveland Clinic CompreCare, and to improve the services offered to physicians and patients, the Cleveland Clinic developed a physician-to-clinic computer link called "Cleveland Clinic CompreLink." It was hoped that the link would make the Cleveland Clinic more responsive. Cleveland Clinic management believed that developing a network for the exchange and storage of information would also provide an important benefit to anyone contracting for services with the Cleveland Clinic or an associated HMO or PPO.

By linking community physicians and the Cleveland Clinic, and exchanging data with community physicians, the Cleveland Clinic believes it would be able to offer employers and other payers data on the outcomes of medical care that would convince such payers that the Cleveland Clinic provides high-quality, effective services at a competitive price. Management also believes that although the Cleveland Clinic needs community physicians, it does not necessarily need close affiliation with community hospitals, as discussed earlier. The link will allow the Cleveland Clinic to maintain close contact directly with physicians.

Strategy

Before starting the program, Cleveland Clinic management came to a number of conclusions:

— They were not interested in supporting a practice management system (i.e., a system in the physician's office that did billing, and maintained accounts receivable and patient records). Hospitals can provide major advantages to physicians who have such systems by transmitting patient data to allow the completion of bills. Since referring physicians do not treat patients at the Cleveland Clinic, the clinic could not offer physicians any benefits in this area.

— Any system should be oriented to the transmission of clinical information, since the Cleveland Clinic could offer such information to the physician and increase its value by offering clinical expertise.

— Legal counsel for the clinic felt that no computer donations to physicians should be made since it could be construed as a reward for referrals.

After considerable searching and evaluation, the IMS 2000 system offered by Integrated Medical Systems, Inc., of Golden, Colorado, was selected. The IMS system offers to the physician an IBM-compatible workstation with a hard disk and modem that has added features. Patient acquisition devices can be attached to allow data from stress ECG, ambulatory blood pressure, Holter monitoring, and pulmonary function tests to be stored and transmitted.

Although the hardware and software were important, management believed that the internal issues involved in establishing the link were the most important and the most difficult. The size of the Cleveland Clinic made it difficult to educate physicians and staff about the nature and purpose of CompreLink, and to ensure a high level of service to physicians.

The Pilot Project

A three-month pilot project was begun in October 1987. Letters were mailed to 1,000 affiliate physicians asking them if they were interested in a computer link to the Cleveland Clinic. Approximately 300 replied they were interested, and 120 actually came to an explanation and demonstration of the link. Physicians, their office staff, or both completed a survey at the demonstration to assess their interest.

Twenty-two sites (with a total of 65 physicians) were selected from this group. The Cleveland Clinic tried to select a group representative of the Cleveland Clinic's referring physicians, including a mix of solo and group practice physicians, specialists and primary care physicians, some using computers and others who did not, physicians who referred to different departments within the Cleveland Clinic, and physicians from various geographic areas serviced by the Cleveland Clinic.

The medical director of CompreLink wrote to the remaining physicians telling them that they would have an opportunity to develop a computer link after the completion of the pilot. A subset of five physician offices was selected for a pilot of the pulmonary function patient acquisition device and software.

All physicians received an IBM-compatible PC with a hard disk and modem. Communications, word processing, electronic drug reference, health risk appraisal, and diet/nutrition/exercise patient education software were included on their hard disks.

To receive a report on their health risks (for example, risk of heart disease) or recommendations on diet, nutrition, or exercise, patients completed questionnaires. The data were entered into the computer, which produced a report. Physicians could choose whether or not to charge for this service.

The functions performed by the CompreLink system itself included the following:

— Pulmonary function data, which could be read by physicians at the Cleveland Clinic who have agreed to provide an overread of the data, can be transmitted.

— Requests for scheduling outpatient services can be made, with an acknowledgment transmitted back upon confirmation. If an IMS practice management system is being used, the physician's office can transmit the necessary patient data without reentering it.

— An update on a patient's treatment can be requested and received.

— A notification of admission to the hospital is sent to the referring physician.

— Results are reported to the referring physician, including a discharge summary and test results from selected departments.

Evaluation of the Pilot

The system was operational at all sites by December 1987. At the end of the pilot in March 1988, use of the system was examined. The message function proved to be extremely popular. There were few messages sent between physicians; most messages were to and from the Cleveland Clinic's staff and departments.

Physicians did use the scheduling functions available in this system, but their use of the drug reference data base was small. Although staff could not measure the extent to which physicians had used the risk appraisal software and patient education modules included with the system, they believed that use of these components was small as well.

An analysis comparing referrals in the two years prior to the pilot to referrals during the pilot period showed an average of four new referrals per site over a six-month period. On the basis of this information and a survey showing a high level of satisfaction by physicians in the pilot, the Board of Governors voted for full implementation of the CompreLink program, extending the offer to all affiliate physicians.

Marketing and Implementation of CompreLink

A demonstration for interested physicians and their staffs was held in May 1988. The Cleveland Clinic hired physician field representatives in June. Implementation of the CompreLink program began in August 1988.

Pricing

The Cleveland Clinic provides each participating physician with the basic workstation (without the patient acquisition devices), software for communication and support, and maintenance. Physicians are asked to pay for one-third of the cost of this package, which was $35 per month in 1989. They are told that they may terminate the agreement with 90-days notice. Agreements are made for three years, with the expectation that an upgrade of equipment is possible at the end of this period. The physician must also lease a dedicated telephone line for $35 per month from the telephone company.

Physicians can purchase or lease software from IMS that can provide a health risk appraisal and offer advice on exercise/diet/nutrition. An additional charge can be made for each service. Physicians can also acquire patient acquisition devices that can be plugged into the computer provided by the Cleveland Clinic and used to generate revenue from pulmonary function tests, stress ECG, Holter monitoring, and ambulatory blood pressure tests. The clinical tests are done in the physician's office, and the data is not sent to the Cleveland Clinic unless an overread is desired and the clinic's physicians have agreed to provide one (overreads were only available for pulmonary function tests in early 1989). The software provided with the devices produces a report that explains the results. Physicians who use the revenue-generating components of the system can potentially generate net revenues higher than the $70 per month cost of the system.

Relationship with the Vendor

Physicians may also buy the equipment, patient acquisition devices, and a practice management system (for $3,000–7,000 in 1989) directly from IMS. The Cleveland Clinic was the alpha (developmental) site for the IMS 2000 system. IMS hired two full-time equivalent staff to be on-site during the pilot doing training, installation, and support. IMS's local field representatives visit physicians at the request of a CompreCare field representative who has found through discussions with physicians that they wish to purchase software and patient acquisition devices directly from IMS.

Cost

The Cleveland Clinic purchases $4,000 in hardware and communications software for each site from IMS. It then sells the system to a leasing company, which leases it back to the Cleveland Clinic for $127 per month.

The price paid to IMS during the first year depended on volume. If at least 400 sites were linked at the end of the first year, the price remained the same. If the number was less, the Cleveland Clinic agreed to pay a penalty, with the amount determined by how many sites were linked.

Staffing

Cleveland Clinic CompreCare and CompreLink are staffed by the Office of Physician Liaison and Alumni Affairs within the Division of Public Affairs and Corporate Development. Under the director of Physician Liaison and Alumni Affairs is a Medical Service manager. The Medical Service representatives, who report to her, support both the CompreCare and CompreLink programs by visiting physician offices to provide information on the program, train staff, and evaluate physician and staff satisfaction.

The Office of Physician Health Affairs is responsible for all strategic efforts of the foundation, including Cleveland Clinic CompreCare. The office is headed by a physician director, who serves as the medical staff contact with affiliate physicians, other clinics, and hospitals. He also receives all complaints from CompreCare affiliate physicians and is responsible for communicating with the chairman of the department involved, and back to the referring physician. The chairman of each department also gets a copy of any complaints. Another physician acts as medical director for this office. His primary responsibility is for the CompreLink project.

Participant Selection

Any physician who has joined CompreCare can also join CompreLink. CompreLink is available to any physician in the Cleveland Clinic's local and regional market areas.

Promotion

A letter was sent to all CompreCare affiliate physicians inviting them and their office managers to attend an "expo" in May 1988 and see a demonstration of the CompreLink system. Two hundred and fifty people attended. Since then, promotion has been through the Cleveland Clinic CompreCare field representatives.

The field representatives do not try to visit every CompreCare physician to explain and demonstrate CompreLink since the distances to outlying physicians in the region are great and the Cleveland Clinic wants to target certain physicians. The criteria for targeting physicians include whether the physician is in the local market area (since training and support are easier), whether the physician is currently a high user of the clinic's services, and the potential number of future referrals as indicated by the trend since the physician became a CompreCare affiliate.

At the first visit to a high-priority physician, the field representative explains the components of the CompreCare program to the office manager and the physician, including a verbal description of CompreLink. They actively promote CompreLink and attempt to arrange a demonstration for both office staff and physicians based on the priority they assign to the site. The CompreCare physician field representatives make at least one visit per quarter to a CompreLink physician's office.

Current Procedures and Functions for CompreLink

Hardware and Software

The Cleveland Clinic strategy has been to use standard PC-compatible hardware, offering physicians the potential to use a wide variety of other software packages. The system has a flag that shows that a message is waiting, allowing office staff to use the computer for multiple purposes.

The system uses a front-end processor rather than terminal emulation software. This means that the user sees screens that have been custom designed for physician offices, rather than what a user of the clinic's computer system would see at a Cleveland Clinic facility. Thus, physicians and office staff do not have to learn a new vocabulary or be confronted with screens with irrelevant information on them.

Support

Field representatives for IMS are responsible for supporting the hardware, software, and data bases provided under an agreement with the Cleveland Clinic. Questions or problems concerning the computer hardware or software can be directed to IMS via a toll-free number.

Physicians or office staff who have a question or problem regarding CompreLink or the Cleveland Clinic can send a message to their Medical Service representative or Cleveland Clinic Affiliate Services. CompreLink staff at the Cleveland Clinic receive requests for information on patient progress and any requests for assistance. A central scheduling office receives requests for, and schedules, appointments. The cardiology and orthopedics departments do their own scheduling.

A key operator and a backup operator from each site are trained during a one-day session at the Cleveland Clinic by both CompreLink and IMS staff. The morning is devoted to the hardware and communications software, and the afternoon to teaching word processing.

Security

The CompreLink software runs on a dedicated MicroVax computer. Since sites are not connected to the Cleveland Clinic mainframe, there is no danger of unauthorized entry, a concern of Cleveland Clinic physicians. Schedulers look at two terminals when making an appointment, one connected to the MicroVax and the other to the Cleveland Clinic mainframe. No passwords or identification numbers are required to use the CompreLink system.

Functions

In addition to the functions available to pilot study sites listed earlier, CompreLink allows physicians and their staffs to

— request drug information from a Cleveland Clinic staff pharmacist at the Cleveland Clinic Drug Information Center

— request information on Cancer Center programs (the Cancer Center uses CompreLink to announce calls for clinical trials, and an affiliate physician could then ask that a patient participate)

— request pamphlets and information for patients from the Cleveland Clinic Patient Information Department

— register for continuing medical education courses

— receive an announcement when one of their patients is admitted as an inpatient that includes the room and telephone numbers

— receive overreads of neuropsychiatric tests

— receive reference lab results (the Cleveland Clinic performs rare and difficult tests for physicians)

Included in the system is a network directory that lists the names and addresses of all Cleveland Clinic departments and CompreCare affiliate physicians accessible via CompreLink. A user can simply select the appropriate name to be entered into a message. The CompreLink system will then send the message to the appropriate location. Physicians can therefore send messages to each other, as well as to the Cleveland Clinic.

The system shows if a message has been read. The system does not automatically delete any message. Someone must manually delete a message, presumably after determining if all appropriate actions have been taken.

A file can be attached to a message, for example, a file containing a patient's medical history or diagnostic test results. The file must reside on the hard disk or a diskette in the computer's disk drive. The system includes a word processor for creating files.

Appendix I shows the screens (i.e., what appears on the screen of the monitor) used to create and send a message on CompreLink.

Evaluation of CompreLink

Evaluation Plan

Ad hoc reports are produced manually three to four times a year to compare referrals that month by CompreLink physicians to the previous year. The additional referrals are multiplied by a standard revenue per referral (no distinction to be made between outpatient and inpatient) to determine additional revenue.

A report could be prepared that used data on referrals from the CompreLink system, but management believes it would be less accurate. Additional referrals may occur that were not made through CompreLink's scheduling function. If a physician uses the general message function, the referral would not be counted. The cardiology and orthopedics departments make their own appointments. When they are called on the phone by a CompreLink site, they may not record the appointment as one from a CompreLink physician. Patients also call the Cleveland Clinic directly, and do not mention the name of the referring physician.

The CompreLink system cannot tabulate the number of referrals by user password to determine which specific individual (for example, the physician or office manager) sent the message since no passwords are used. The number of times a reference data base has been accessed also cannot be determined. The system can tabulate the number of messages sent, but not the specific task performed, for example, a health information request or a patient update request.

Since the risk appraisal and nutrition assessment software reside on the user's hard disk, the Cleveland Clinic also has no way of determining how often these are used. Nor can the Cleveland Clinic determine the number of times a clinical test was performed in offices that have patient acquisition devices.

Field representatives survey physicians and office staff about their satisfaction with services, including the CompreLink system, during their quarterly site visits. No surveys or interviews are conducted with patients to determine their level of satisfaction with services provided over the CompreLink system.

Results

In early 1989, there were approximately 2,000 messages per month sent by the 40 sites on the link. The monthly report for September 1988 showed an average of 3.8 referrals per site for that month. No attempt has been made since the pilot to compare the number of referrals before and after the installation of the link.

Interviews with physicians suggested that they were pleased with the results. One physician described how the processing of referrals had changed with the CompreLink system. The physician believed that the patient might have a parathyroid tumor. There were no local physicians that he wished to refer the patient to for this problem. He was not sure whether the patient should see a surgeon or an endocrinologist. In the past, he would have looked in the Cleveland Clinic directory and guessed which physician might treat the patient. Instead, he sent a message over CompreLink to affiliate services, where a Cleveland Clinic staff member researched the problem and suggested that the patient be referred to a specific endocrinologist. This saved the patient a trip since the physician could have made a referral to a surgeon if the link was not in place.

Another physician reported that CompreLink helped him and his partners stay close to the patient. They make an extra effort to provide a high level of service, which includes quickly scheduling patients for appointments and quickly reporting test results. This physician had already agreed to be a site for a physician-to-hospital link with the local hospital. CompreLink allowed the group to provide a similar level of service to their patients seen at the Cleveland Clinic. They could look at whether services had been scheduled and provided, and help the patient resolve problems. They viewed the patient update function as very important since it assured that information would be available whenever the patient was seen at their office.

Interviews detected some problems with the scheduling system also. A physician who made a referral to a specialist later received a call from a resident at the Cleveland Clinic asking him about the patient, who had been admitted to the Cleveland Clinic. The physician had not been informed of the admission, even though he was a CompreCare affiliate and used CompreLink. The CompreLink system did not at that time have automatic admission notification. Physicians were expected to use the patient update function, which they would not do unless they knew the patient had been admitted. The physician felt that he had not been adequately informed.

On the other hand, the physician admitted that he did not use the patient update function because Cleveland Clinic specialists usually sent a letter after a referral within a week, which was usually before the patient was seen again. While the traditional manual system provides a backup, it may also deter a physician from continually using CompreLink to obtain information, resulting in some information never being seen.

Another physician reported that a message was sent using CompreLink requesting an appointment for a test from a department that operated its own scheduling system. There was no response, and after three days of calls and messages, the physician gave up and sent the patient elsewhere. This illustrates the problems raised by decentralized scheduling, which makes it more difficult for CompreLink staff to assure good service, especially when busy departments are involved.

On the other hand, the physician had not sent a message to his CompreCare service representative or to the director of Physician Health Affairs, who serves as the focal point for physician complaints and concerns. Complaints are tracked until they are investigated and a response made.

Growth of CompreLink

An offer to join CompreLink was made to the 3,000 CompreCare physicians through a newsletter item in August 1988. As of January 1989, 40 sites with

127 physicians were using CompreLink. The increase in the number of physician offices that were linked was less than expected by management.

A number of explanations were offered by Cleveland Clinic management and staff. One explanation was that the physicians were cautious about accepting an offer of assistance without fully understanding the motives of the Cleveland Clinic. Each physician's office was being given $4,000 in hardware and software at a very low cost. The Cleveland Clinic paid $127 per month for a hardware and software lease. Physicians were required to pay a $35 a month hardware and software maintenance and support fee, as well as $35 a month for a dedicated telephone line. Some physicians viewed this offer with suspicion, asking why the Cleveland Clinic would do this and what the Cleveland Clinic wanted. Other physicians voiced the opinion that if the link benefited the Cleveland Clinic, it should bear all of the costs.

Some of the field representatives reported that while physicians were interested in the link, they met opposition from their office staff who did not want to use a computer. Some physicians voiced the opinion that although the system was not too expensive, the cost was not justified because of the low volume of referrals they made to the Cleveland Clinic.

Although there were some exceptions, Cleveland Clinic staff believed that older physicians were not interested in the link because they did not want to change their current procedures within a few years of retirement. They received a much more enthusiastic response from younger physicians who believed that use of the computer in their medical practice was essential.

Some physicians reported being deceived by computer sales personnel who sold them inappropriate computer hardware and software. This experience left the physicians wary of any computer application they had to pay for.

Another possible explanation was the relatively small number of functions that could be performed over the link. The Cleveland Clinic had not offered practice management software as part of the package. It was also recognized that the Cleveland Clinic did not possess data needed by the referring physician for billing, since referring physicians provided no services to patients in Cleveland Clinic facilities. Although they believed that the link offered important services, the functions that could be performed were quite limited.

Because of the size of the Cleveland Clinic and the other tasks that had to be accomplished, Cleveland Clinic management and CompreLink staff did not have time during the pilot and implementation stages to educate many Cleveland Clinic staff and physicians concerning the goals of CompreLink and what they were expected to do. This had an impact on the system in several ways. Departments did not always use CompreLink to send back the results of a test or consultation. Mail and telephone contact were used. Second, Cleveland Clinic physicians did not become advocates for CompreLink when they dealt with local and regional referral physicians.

Management plans in the future to engage in much more internal marketing. More Cleveland Clinic physicians and staff will be trained. Cleveland Clinic physicians will be asked to prioritize local and regional physicians as targets for CompreLink, and to call those physicians to educate them about the value and need for CompreLink.

In order to develop a larger number of sites in a shorter period of time, Cleveland Clinic staff had not actively marketed the ability of the IMS hardware to collect and transmit pulmonary function tests. A physician who performs such tests would be able to generate additional revenue and would have the ability to transmit results to pulmonary specialists at the Cleveland Clinic. However, using the CompreLink system for this function requires the purchase of a $4,000 pulmonary function device that provides an interface to the microcomputer. Although physicians might be able to quickly generate the revenue required to pay for this system, it was an additional capital expense for physicians.

Some physicians also were not interested in using the revenue-generating software that came with the system during the pilot. If the physician did not want to use the system to generate revenue from health risk appraisal and diet/exercise/nutrition assessment and education, the modest monthly cost of CompreLink was an additional cost of operating the practice.

Since the ability of the IMS system to perform and transmit clinical tests was a major factor in its selection and could make the link financially attractive to physicians, the experience of the Cleveland Clinic with this function will be examined in greater detail.

The Importance of Clinical Testing Capabilities

The CompreLink system allows for the transmission of data from pulmonary function tests to the Cleveland Clinic, where physicians can do an overread (a second reading and interpretation of the data). The charge in 1989 was $25. In addition, the IMS 2000 system has the capability to carry out and transmit stress ECG, Holter monitoring, and ambulatory blood pressure tests. Physicians can purchase the patient acquisition devices from IMS to perform these three tests, but the Cleveland Clinic does not perform overreads of the results.

The ability to perform these tests and transmit the results to the Cleveland Clinic has certain potential benefits for the referring physician, the patient, and the Cleveland Clinic:

— The physician can take advantage of expertise at the Cleveland Clinic to verify an interpretation.

— Physicians can demonstrate to patients that they use the latest computer-based equipment and are backed up by the Cleveland Clinic.

— The physician can generate additional revenue by performing tests in the office, rather than referring the patient elsewhere.

— The patient can receive the added benefit of the confirmation of an interpretation by a specialist.

— The Cleveland Clinic can offer support to its referring physicians, possibly leading to greater loyalty.

— The Cleveland Clinic may receive additional referrals that might otherwise go to a local specialist.

In order for significant benefits to be realized, a number of assumptions must be correct for more than a few patients:

— The physician is interested in an overread of a test rather than a consultation with a specialist that involves an evaluation of all the data and actually examining the patient.

— An overread is not easily available locally.

— Physicians wish to do the test in their offices and need new or replacement equipment.

Interviews with a few physicians suggest that these assumptions may not always be true and need to be carefully questioned.

The Cleveland Clinic serves its referring physicians by providing the expertise of specialists to treat patients whose problems are relatively rare or complex. Emphasis is placed on physician-to-physician contacts, and few patients come to the Cleveland Clinic just for a medical procedure.

Community hospitals and physicians' offices are now capable of performing most of the procedures available at the Cleveland Clinic. Referring physicians may have very few patients for whom a timely overread is needed and cannot be obtained locally. If the problem is neither rare nor complex (for example, asthma, high blood pressure or a mild arrhythmia), the physician may treat the problem or want the patient to be treated locally. However, a referring physician may still want a confirmation from a Cleveland Clinic specialist for legal reasons, for example, when rendering a judgment on a patient's level of disability that could be challenged in the courts.

Computer-based testing can also free the physician from the need to use a specialist (while, ironically, making data transmission easier). The software used to process the results of a Holter test dissects or decomposes the results and provides the physician with a comparison of each component to preset guidelines. The results are available immediately since the cartridges do not have to be sent away. The software for the pulmonary function tests highlights abnormal results.

Although the ability to obtain additional revenue by performing clinical tests is a potential advantage for physicians, their willingness to purchase the IMS patient acquisition devices depends on their perception of the costs and benefits of these devices in comparison with IMS's competitors. There are a number of reasons why physicians might not purchase the patient acquisition devices:

— They already have the equipment and do not want to replace it.

— They judge a stand-alone device to be superior.

— They only wish to perform one test, so the economic advantage of using a single computer for multiple tests is reduced.

— They are not dissatisfied with their current source.

— They do not wish to antagonize a current source.

— They may not want to take the responsibility for performing the tests.

— They perceive themselves to be too busy to get involved.

— They are afraid of using a computer.

Cleveland Clinic management has not actively promoted the use of patient acquisition devices and overreads. Physicians in five of the pilot sites were given the devices; other physicians must now pay for them. Management is concerned that physicians will see the cost of the patient acquisition devices as a cost of participating in the link, reducing the number of physicians who join.

Internal Reaction to Clinical Testing

In order for referring physicians to receive the benefits of an overread, Cleveland Clinic physicians have to be willing to accept the process and provide interpretations in a timely manner. During the pilot, only pulmonary function tests were transmitted. Cleveland Clinic pulmonary specialists were initially concerned about the quality of the data. A Cleveland Clinic respiratory therapist was hired by IMS as their field representative. This individual trained the office staff who would perform the tests during a two-day session at the Cleveland Clinic and was present when they performed the first one at the physician's office. This reduced the concern of the Cleveland Clinic physicians.

Although referring physicians were told that they would receive a timely overread, no exact standard or norm was given, nor was one obtained from the Cleveland Clinic physicians who do the interpretations. Cleveland Clinic management has not sought agreement with other departments to perform overreads of other tests because of a concern that timely service would not be provided. There is no formal procedure for tracking the speed with which an overread is provided. The system does not track the request for an overread from the time a request is made until the interpretation is sent out.

No research has been carried out to determine the number of physicians who perceive the benefits of clinical testing to be high, who view the costs of CompreLink to be easily offset by its capability to produce additional revenue, and who would desire overreads. Until these data are available, it is not clear how important the availability of overreads for other tests is to the success of CompreLink.

Future Development

Competition from Other Systems

Cleveland Clinic CompreLink faces competition from physician-to-hospital computer links offered by community hospitals. It faces potential competition from other regional referral centers (for example, the Mayo Clinic, Henry Ford Hospital, and the University of Michigan Hospitals) that could offer a similar service. Cleveland Clinic management has no information on their plans, but these institutions have the same needs and adequate resources.

Three community hospitals have developed, or are developing, a link. One of the links incorporates a practice management system that does patient billing. The operator looks at a split screen that shows hospital data next to the physician's own billing form. Data can be moved directly from the hospital's computer into such forms. Although this system in no way duplicates CompreLink, some physicians may be unwilling to pay the costs of both systems.

On the other hand, the immediate benefits of connecting to the local hospital may induce more physicians to make the investment in hardware and telephone lines. If the CompreLink software can reside on the same computer and switching is easy, the presence of these local systems could stimulate the growth of CompreLink.

Early in 1989, the head of pediatrics at a hospital in the region asked the Cleveland Clinic to link his department to CompreLink to allow him to communicate with pediatricians in his local community and with the children's hospital being developed at the Cleveland Clinic. Management feels this could become an alternative strategy for meeting the needs of physicians while discussions about the designation of hub hospitals continue. A reference lab also approached the clinic early in 1989 to ask if it could be linked, since this would speed up the transmission of lab results.

Enhancements

Management planned to add the following enhancements to CompreLink in 1989:

— the reference data bases for poisons, drugs, capsule and tablet identification, and emergency medicine offered by Micromedex, Inc., of Denver, Colorado

— ECAT, a catalog of continuing medical education courses and patient education seminars and brochures that includes the capability to enter a registration (ECAT is offered by the University of Alabama, Birmingham)

— a link to the Cleveland Clinic IBM mainframe, which would allow messages to be sent to any department at the Cleveland Clinic not already connected to CompreLink

The Cleveland Clinic intends to hire a registered nurse to ensure that information on the services provided to the patients of CompreCare physicians goes out quickly—either immediately over CompreLink, or in the mails the same day for sites that are not linked. This will include postoperative notes, which will be generated in the operating room. The Cleveland Clinic also intends to hire a full-time technical person to assist with CompreLink.

Management is still considering whether to add the capability to transmit stress ECG and Holter monitoring tests if the physician purchases the necessary patient acquisition device(s).

The survey undertaken to evaluate the pilot showed that physicians wanted the ability to do medical literature searches and electronic claims submission. Management is considering the addition of both capabilities.

Fax

In the future, the use of fax transmission may also emerge as a technology competing with data transmission by computer. Although fax machines do not offer all the advantages of a computer, they can perform many other functions in an office, in addition to transmitting test results. They are also simple and easy to use.

Management believes that providing a fax machine to physicians, and developing the procedures for accepting fax transmissions to perform functions now done with CompreLink, may be necessary to induce some physicians to join CompreLink.

Those physicians who have already purchased fax machines for transmitting text between offices and to a hospital or lab can easily use these machines to communicate with the Cleveland Clinic. Those who have not purchased one can justify the purchase on the basis of the multiple capabilities of the machine for physician-to-physician and physician-to-hospital or lab communications.

Although a fax machine is a combination of a microprocessor, memory, modem, and printer, it is not viewed as a computer, producing the anxiety that computers produce. It can also transmit handwritten notes and records that make up a substantial part of a patient's medical record.

The danger of encouraging the use of fax is that it may become more difficult to convince physicians that computer-to-computer transmission offers substantial additional advantages.

Support for CompreLink

Management believes that a physician-to-hospital computer link is a good long-term strategy that will support alliances with referring physicians, help in the development of managed care options such as PPOs, and improve the flow of information needed to provide high-quality care. It will help the Cleveland Clinic demonstrate to employers that it can manage medical care and track both utilization and outcomes for a widely dispersed population. Support for CompreLink remains strong, and the Cleveland Clinic is now looking for ways to increase the number of physicians using the link.

Notes

1. W. R. Gombeski, Jr., C. E. Stone, and F. J. Weaver, "Improving Services through a Professional Shopper Program," *Journal of Health Care Marketing* 6, no. 3 (1986): 64–68.
2. W. R. Gombeski, Jr., G. W. Fay, K. R. Niedzielski, and F. J. Weaver, "Evaluating Promotional Strategy Effectiveness for a Health Care Organization," *Journal of Business Research* 17, no. 1 (August 1988): 81–90.

12.

Samaritan Health Services' Development of a Hospital-to-Physician Computer Link

Introduction

Samaritan Health Services (SHS) is a multihospital corporation with head-quarters in Phoenix, Arizona. Samaritan Health Services owns, leases, or sponsors seven hospitals with a total of 1,596 beds and manages under contract two other hospitals with a total of 50 beds. The four hospitals with over 200 beds each are all located in the Phoenix metropolitan area. They had 30 percent of the total hospital discharges during the first half of 1988 (see Table 12.1). Its largest hospital is 648-bed Good Samaritan Medical Center, a teaching facility located in downtown Phoenix.

From October 1986 to May 1987, Samaritan Health Services conducted a $150,000 pilot project, which linked 12 sites (with 60 physicians) to SHS's central data-processing center located in its corporate headquarters, adjacent to Good Samaritan Medical Center. Based on the success of the pilot, it began in November 1988 to offer a physician-to-hospital computer link to a larger group of physicians.

This case was prepared by Roger Kropf, Ph.D., for publication and use in classroom discussion, rather than to illustrate either effective or ineffective handling of an administrative situation. The author wishes to thank the following Samaritan Health Services managers for their generous support in the preparation of this case: Clarence Teng, President; Charles C. Emery, Jr., Vice-President of Information Services; and Cheryl Clancy, R.N., Manager of the Pulse System.

Table 12.1   Maricopa County Hospital Utilization, First Half 1988

Hospital	Total Discharges	Days	Average LOS	Occupancy (%)	Births
Boswell	6,854	51,194	7.5	79.2%	0
Chandler Regional	3,838	15,597	4.1	66.6	578
Del E. Webb Memorial	682	5,816	8.5	15.7	0
*Desert Samaritan	12,750	54,834	4.3	76.1	2,545
*Good Samaritan Medical Center	17,110	94,336	5.5	72.8	2,809
Humana Deer Valley	3,037	12,651	4.2	45.9	406
Humana Phoenix	4,121	26,243	6.4	45.3	186
John C. Lincoln	5,544	29,830	5.4	56.1	472
Maricopa Medical Center	12,357	63,684	5.2	52.8	2,728
*Maryvale Samaritan	5,444	26,743	4.9	53.9	690
Mesa General	2,957	12,174	4.1	54.5	439
Mesa Lutheran	6,621	35,139	5.3	49.0	768
Phoenix Baptist	5,406	28,078	5.2	61.4	592
Phoenix Community	993	4,324	4.4	30.0	156
Phoenix General	2,530	16,060	6.3	31.0	0
Phoenix General Deer Valley	1,523	5,615	3.7	28.5	217
Phoenix Memorial	4,323	17,087	4.0	42.1	936
Scottsdale Memorial	8,130	43,839	5.4	69.0	678
Scottsdale Memorial North	3,334	14,766	4.4	70.6	465
St. Josephs Phoenix	15,794	95,774	6.1	75.8	2,331
St. Luke	2,890	18,834	6.5	46.8	0
Tempe St. Luke	1,934	7,956	4.1	38.2	193
*Thunderbird Samaritan	6,027	25,682	4.3	62.2	925
Valley Lutheran	2,998	19,068	6.4	87.3	0
Valley View	986	7,465	7.6	39.4	0
Totals	138,183	732,789	5.3	58.2	18,114

*Samaritan Health Services Hospital.
Source: Samaritan Health Services, *Market Assessment and Performance Indicators 1989*, p. CP-33.
Reprinted by permission.

SHS wanted to reward loyal physicians and influence physicians who split admissions. The environment in Phoenix is one in which physicians maintain multiple hospital affiliations and will change the hospitals they use quickly. SHS felt it could not ignore its loyal physicians and could reward them by offering access to its data bases at a relatively low cost.

SHS also wanted the link to improve communications with purchasers such as employers, HMOs, and PPOs. The link would allow purchasers to receive information on admissions and the course of treatment being offered, and would allow SHS to receive authorization for treatment faster and to determine patient eligibility under various insurance and payment plans.

The Pilot Project

Administrators from each SHS Phoenix-area hospital recommended physicians for inclusion in the pilot project. Eleven physician offices and one HMO volunteered. The HMO was a major customer of SHS and provided SHS with 10–15 percent of its patients. Only one of the HMO's sites, with 42 physicians, was linked.

The 11 other sites had from one to seven physicians. The specialties (with the number of physicians in parentheses) included pediatrics (4), anesthesiology (7), internal medicine/chest diseases (4), internal medicine/pulmonary (1), internal medicine/gastroenterology (3), two other internal medicine groups (5 and 2), family practice/OB/GYN (2), OB/GYN (4), high-risk OB (4), and surgery (1).

The functions that physicians and their staffs could perform during the pilot included admission/account history inquiry, census (list of patients in the hospital and their locations), display orders, demographic/insurance inquiry, lab results inquiry, medical record abstract inquiry, and patient inquiry. (A more detailed description of these functions is found later in this case.)

Of the seven offices with computer systems, four were not IBM-compatible. The physicians were lent the hardware and software they needed at no charge. Hardware and software were selected that allowed each site to emulate a terminal connected to SHS's main computer. The physicians and their staffs could then perform a limited number of functions as if they were in the hospital itself. Commands were entered using a light pen.

Evaluation of the Pilot

Data were collected on the use of the system by the computer and through personal interviews at the conclusion of the pilot project. The number of times each function was used during the month of April 1987 is shown in Table 12.2.

When respondents were asked to describe the benefits of the system, 76 percent said that it increased their efficiency by reducing the number of telephone calls to the hospital. When asked if they were willing to continue to commit resources to the system, 80 percent said yes.

Respondents also made recommendations for future enhancements. However, with the exception of improvements in how the patient census was displayed (18 percent wanted improvements), less than 10 percent of respondents favored any particular improvement. For example, 5 percent wanted transcribed reports displayed. This suggested either that there were not major critical needs that respondents believed the system could meet or that respondents had difficulty understanding what the system could or could not do, and the benefits that might result.

Table 12.2   Use of Functions on SHS's Computer Link in April 1987

Function	Frequency	Percent Utilization
Account history	30	4%
Census	468	59%
Demographic/insurance	166	21%
Display orders	19	2%
Help	13	2%
Lab results	29	3%
Medical record abstract	13	2%
Patient inquiry	58	7%
Total	796	100%

At the end of the pilot, SHS's management and board agreed that full implementation should be the next step, with a goal of 40 sites at the end of the first year, increasing by 40 in the second year, 40 in the third year, and 12 in the fourth year. This would result in a total of 132 sites. Beyond that, additional hardware would have to be added to SHS's mainframe computer.

Development of a Business Plan

SHS management prepared a business plan for a physician-to-hospital link in 1988 to support a decision on whether to proceed with full implementation. The sections that follow summarize the contents of that plan.

Market Analysis

Potential customers

Physicians.   SHS management believed that physicians were experiencing many of the same competitive threats as hospitals. Physician practices were being squeezed by a potential 70,000-physician surplus by 1990, Medicare cutbacks for physician services, and affiliations with alternative delivery systems. Just as hospitals were offering more services that were once offered only in medical offices, large clinics were offering services previously offered only by hospital facilities.

The key issues of concern to physicians were believed to be increased competition for patients, patient visits trending down, more complex office administration, more demanding health care consumers, and anticipations that various forms of physician fee constraints would be implemented and that new forms of health care delivery would threaten the survival of their professional way of life.

Consequently, an opportunity existed for hospitals and physicians to combine talents, strengths, and resources in a mutually beneficial relationship to support a health care delivery system that could provide a full spectrum of services to target markets. SHS management believed that one way of achieving this was through a physician-to-hospital computer link.

Physician interest was expected to vary depending on specialty, group affiliation, practice patterns, and level of automation. The pilot project and research literature yielded information about the benefits a computer network could provide to physicians: Convenience and efficiency were those most frequently mentioned. The hospital link would also improve physician cash flow by making available insurance information from the hospital, increase physician productivity by allowing patient location and test results review before making rounds, and streamline office procedures by reducing telephone calls to the hospital through preadmission of patients.

Physicians were also believed to be interested in office automation. However, a survey conducted by the Maricopa Medical Foundation for Medical Care (Phoenix is located in Maricopa County) showed that fewer than 50 percent of all physician offices used an automated practice management system or electronic claims program. Lack of knowledge about hardware, software, and communications were significant barriers to automation. Physicians were justifiably wary of vendors and had suggested that assistance would be beneficial in the evaluation and selection of office systems. SHS Information Services had personnel with experience in system analysis and selection, and could therefore provide a valuable service to physicians by making these existing resources available.

Physicians had expressed an interest in networking with SHS. Approximately 25 percent of the medical offices in the Phoenix area had computers that were capable of communicating with the SHS system if minor hardware and software enhancements were made.

Enhancements to the computer network would allow physicians to communicate with other SHS entities such as Visiting Nurse Service (VNS) and Samaritan Home Health Stores. It would also help foster relationships between hospital-based specialists and regional physicians, at first by allowing regional physicians to access information about their patients in SHS Phoenix-area facilities. Later, it could be used to support clinical outreach programs.

Managed care plans.   Current hospital census information was necessary for managed care plans to monitor the activities of physicians and hospitals and perform utilization review functions, key factors determining the profitability of managed care plans. Verification of insurance, time consuming for both insurers and providers, could be streamlined with the system.

Employers.   The essence of marketing to employers was believed to be the development of quality, price-competitive packages of health services. Because of the effect of health care costs on their income statements, most large employers with comprehensive health care programs were becoming price elastic in their selection of health care providers.

Through analysis of past and recent experience for a given employer, the system would be capable of projecting health care usage patterns and alerting employers to negative trends. Where reporting to state and federal agencies on employee health and safety was required, employer-level reporting would be a valuable added benefit. The Pulse system would also allow employers to monitor use of facilities and providers.

Market size

To estimate the potential size of the network, data from the Arizona Department of Health Services and hospital medical staff files were analyzed. There were approximately 2,270 physicians with staff privileges at SHS Phoenix-area facilities in 1988. However, 498 of these physicians accounted for 80 percent of the admissions to those SHS facilities. The office locations of these key admitters were spread over a wide geographical area, but some were clustered in office buildings close to the hospitals. There were 61 regional (i.e., outside of the Phoenix area) physicians, 10 HMOs, and 15 PPOs.

If all of these individuals and organizations were participating in the network, there would be approximately 584 installations. This was approximately the size of the terminal network that supported Good Samaritan Medical Center. However, the physicians would generate far less activity and demand on computer resources than the hospital.

Competitors

St. Joseph's Hospital and Medical Center was the first hospital in Phoenix to attempt to establish a hospital-to-physician computer link. It contracted in 1988 with the San Diego consulting firm of Magliaro and McHaney to develop a separate company called Arizona Health Sources.

SHS management believed that St. Joseph's invested over $4 million in the project. The marketing strategy selected was to provide, free of charge, a system consisting of an IBM PC, the Doctor's Office Manager practice management system, and the promise of networking in the future. Computers were given to physicians in 200 sites.

St. Joseph's Physician Computer Network was targeted toward the primary care doctors; specialists were to be added later as needed. St. Joseph's concept was to develop a separate corporation to manage the network and to act as a "marketing arm" for the physicians in the network.

However, St. Joseph's was unable to establish communications between the hospital and participants in the network. St. Joseph's did not have a hospital ADT (Admission, Discharge, Transfer) or lab system in place that could be linked. SHS management believed the network could become functional with a nominal investment and a significant, coordinated effort by St. Joseph's management.

SHS management believed that, as of early 1989, many physicians who had received a system from St. Joseph's were not using it to communicate with that hospital, and that some had not installed and used the practice management system they were given. Any of these physicians could easily use SHS's system if given the appropriate software, at little cost to SHS.

Phoenix Baptist Hospital hired a new vice-president of Information Services in 1988. This individual was instrumental in developing the American Hospital Supply (now Baxter) computer network for purchasing. Given his expertise with networking, combined with the maturity of the Phoenix Baptist computer system, this hospital would have an advantage should it decide to establish a network. Baptist, however, was believed to lack the financial resources to develop a link.

The Mayo Clinic presented a competitive threat because of the large number of Mayo alumni residing in Arizona and the institution's reputation for clinical integration. The Mayo Clinic used the CyCare system. CyCare had long been a leader in the ambulatory systems market and had recently entered the hospital systems market. In 1985, it moved its headquarters to Phoenix. CyCare had developed a networking product, which the Mayo Clinic could install rapidly if it decided to establish a network.

SHS management believed that SHS had more information that could be offered through the link than its competitors. However, SHS had not moved quickly to develop the first link in Phoenix. As the second to offer the service, it could meet skepticism that had developed because of the problems with St. Joseph's system.

Objectives

When it began full implementation of the link in 1988, SHS management believed the computer link, referred to as the Pulse system, would expedite the implementation of SHS's marketing strategy in several ways:

1. It would provide physicians and managed care plans with immediate access to computer-based patient information, providing the benefits described earlier.

2. Through selective distribution and access to the link, SHS would provide a direct incentive for physicians, managed care plans, and employers to make SHS the system of choice.

3. Conversely, as access to products, services, and programs through the link increased, the physician relations program would provide a substantial barrier to exit for the physician and a substantial barrier to entrance for the competition.

4. The Pulse system would also provide communications with non-hospital SHS entities, such as Samaritan Health Plan (SHS's IPA HMO), regional facilities, VNS, Samaritan Home Health Stores, Oakmark, and other SHS-related companies, as appropriate.

Generating revenue and covering costs were not identified as primary objectives for the Pulse system. However, the program was expected to achieve a return on investment. Exhibit 12.1 presents part of the financial analysis undertaken to justify the expenditure of funds on the Pulse system.

Weaknesses and Threats

Weaknesses

SHS did not currently have a fully integrated computer system. Until 1985, its four Phoenix-area hospitals developed applications independently of each other. Therefore, the appearance of the systems to the user was substantially different, and the idiosyncrasies of the four systems would make it more difficult to develop applications for the Pulse system. One moderating factor was the standardization of certain key systems (for example, Patient Accounting) undertaken in 1988.

The Pulse system would also develop in an evolutionary manner, which meant that it would have a less revolutionary impact than would be achieved if a complete system was purchased and installed.

Threats

SHS management believed there were several threats to the success of the links. The first was competition. There were at least two competitors that were well positioned to build computer links if adequate resources were dedicated. Other hospital systems might implement a link and use it as a negotiating factor with managed care providers.

Second, because it would be placed in physician offices, the Pulse system was vulnerable. Competitors might begin to offer products that would run on its hardware. If more hospitals dedicated resources to computer links, the practice might evolve into a standard method of communications rather than a unique service that provided SHS a competitive advantage. In addition, physicians might fear that SHS would be able to use the system to monitor their business activities and would therefore be reluctant to participate.

Another threat was the rapidly changing environment in health care. The link had to be flexible and responsive to the needs of physicians, rather than allowing SHS's plans for system implementation to determine how Pulse developed. Information Services was not accustomed to competing in the for-profit sector. Physicians would expect the quality, timely service that they received from other vendors. SHS had to be prepared to provide comparable, if not superior, products and service.

Strategy

Product differentiation

SHS management believed that its major competitive advantage was the hospital's data. By leveraging its existing computer system (i.e., offering access to the wide variety of data already in its computers), SHS could offer physicians a very valuable service at a low cost to SHS. SHS would not integrate the link into a package of services that would include practice management systems and consulting since this would limit access to its data and raise SHS's costs.

SHS sought to develop a product that could support the SHS strategy to continue horizontal and vertical expansion by:

— installing the Pulse system to run on IBM-compatible hardware, which had the greatest potential for acceptance in offices with existing systems

— selecting hardware vendors who could support installations throughout the state of Arizona

— developing alliances with software vendors to increase awareness of the Pulse system in the offices of physicians

Distribution relationships with vendors

SHS chose not to select a single vendor of an office management system for a number of reasons. First, SHS felt that it would be held responsible for the shortcomings of the office management system selected. If receivables increased rather than decreased, for example, physicians might hold SHS responsible and even ask SHS to assist them financially rather than going to a bank to borrow money.

Second, SHS found that 60 percent of the physicians it had targeted as a priority already had a computer, as did 30 percent of all physicians on its medical staffs. These physicians could be antagonistic if SHS selected a single system to support.

Exhibit 12.1   Physician Network Incremental Income and Cash Flow
Statements

Assumptions:

1. Two incremental admissions per installation.
2. SHS absorbs costs of hardware and installation in half of the installations.
3. Physicians provide their own hardware in half of the installations.
4. Physicians absorb costs of telephone line installation at $130 and its maintenance at
   $50/month, as well as insurance to cover replacement costs of hardware if hardware is
   provided by SHS.

Incremental Income Statement

	Projected 1988	Projected 1989	Projected 1990
# of installations	40	80	120
# of incremental admissions	80	160	240
Revenue*	600,000	1,247,999	1,946,888
Reductions	138,000	287,040	447,784
Net revenue	462,000	960,959	1,499,104
Incremental expenses:			
Direct expenses	270,435	562,504	877,506
Salaries			
Manager (1 FTE) and staff (4 FTEs)	157,858	164,172	170,739
Benefits (5 FTEs)	34,729	36,118	37,563
Total salaries and benefits	192,587	200,290	208,302
Supplies	1,800	1,872	1,947
Telecom service at I/S	3,600	7,488	11,681
Maintenance	8,184	26,560	44,145
Depreciation	20,170	37,550	54,930
Total expenses	496,775	836,264	1,198,511
Net incremental income (loss)	(34,775)	124,695	300,593

*Revenue figures have been adjusted to maintain the confidentiality of SHS data.

Continued

Third, 15 vendors of physician office practice systems were active in the
Phoenix area. None had a dominant market share. SHS did not want to
alienate any of the vendors. By not selecting a single vendor, all of the
vendors would be given an interest in supporting the SHS link in order to gain
a competitive advantage in sales to SHS physicians or to meet the competition. SHS could leverage the installed customer base of individual vendors to
provide greater access to SHS data.

Exhibit 12.1 Continued

Financial Assumptions

	Projected 1988	Projected 1989	Projected 1990
I/S Dept. capital budget	$100,850	$86,900	$86,900
Inflation rate (%)	4.00	4.00	4.00
Reductions of revenue (%)	22.96	22.96	22.96
Benefits (%)	22.00	22.00	22.00
Telecom services per unit	360	374	389
# of lines for service	10	20	30

Cash Flow Statement

	Projected 1988	Projected 1989	Projected 1990
Net income (loss)	(34,775)	124,695	300,593
Add:			
Depreciation	20,170	37,550	54,930
Interest	0	0	0
	20,170	37,550	54,930
Less:			
Capital purchases	100,850	86,900	86,900
Net cash flow	(115,455)	75,345	268,623

Source: Samaritan Health Services, *Samaritan Physician Computer Network Business Plan,* IX. Financial Pro Formas, Scenario #4. Reprinted with permission.

From a programmer's point of view, a single vendor strategy would be more desirable since SHS would have to link its computer to only one system. From the perspective of senior management, allowing access to multiple vendors offered the possibility of increasing the rate of growth of the system.

Upon request, SHS staff would provide physicians with information about the features and functions of practice management systems that had an established client base in Phoenix, after which the physicians could make contact with whichever firms they wanted. To become certified as an SHS vendor of practice management software, a vendor would have to agree to work with SHS to develop methods for clients to access SHS's computer. Although they would not be required to do so, some vendors were expected to go ahead and develop programs that interfaced their systems to SHS's, allowing, for example, the downloading of files into the physician's office system. This would be done at no cost to SHS.

Over time, physicians would gain the advantages of practice management systems that had a hospital link (for example, the ability to enter hospital data directly into a physician billing form) but would be free to choose a practice management system based on individual needs and financial capacity.

Pricing

SHS also decided that it would not give physicians computer hardware and software. Although incremental inpatient admissions might justify the costs of installing and supporting a computer network free-of-charge to physicians, relying on this was viewed as undesirable. Physicians might feel this was an attempt to lock them into the use of one hospital. And, although free hardware and software were attractive inducements that would guarantee market penetration, the success of the network depended on actual use of the system. SHS management believed that the connotation of the word "free" was "of little value" and might actually be a deterrent to use.

SHS had loaned equipment to physicians during the pilot. To proceed with full implementation, SHS became a value-added reseller, allowing it to obtain discounts of about 30 percent for physicians. Physicians who wanted and needed hardware were referred to Computerland and IBM. Both would sell just the hardware or bundle it with office management and other software.

The cost to install the hardware and communications software was estimated to be $3,100 per location. If a physician had IBM-compatible hardware, the system could be adapted for $0–500.

SHS Marketing developed a standard offer to be made to all prospective users. There would be no charge if the physician provided the hardware. However, if SHS provided hardware, the user would test the system for six months at no charge. After six months, if the user wanted to continue using it, there would be a charge of approximately $600 per year for five years. This amount would cover the costs of the hardware and service, and some modest contribution to software development costs. It was believed that once the physician or office staff observed the utility of the link, the modest pricing structure proposed would not be a barrier. While this offer was still in effect in April 1989, it had not been used. Physicians have chosen to purchase their own hardware when needed.

Organization and staffing

Management decided that the SHS approach to a link would be substantially different from other hospitals. The link would be organized and managed within SHS, rather than as a separate business entity. In order to assure quality, and minimize cost, the Pulse system would be developed and supported by SHS through contracts with selected microcomputer hardware, software, practice management, and communications vendors. SHS staff responsible for Pulse would coordinate service, monitor the network, and continue to enhance the product.

A staff of four programmer/analysts and a manager was devoted to the implementation of the Pulse system; the manager reported directly to the vice-president of Information Services.

Promotion and participant selection

The SHS Hospital Marketing directors helped develop criteria for physician selection. The dominant criteria was loyalty. Additional factors considered were inpatient and outpatient utilization patterns, revenue generated, office location, medical specialty related to hospital business plan, and other factors such as administrative ratings, committee memberships, and staff relations.

Providing the product to physicians who had not demonstrated a preference for SHS would be risky. This was the strategy adopted by St. Joseph's, with limited success. Physicians who split their practices did so for reasons that might not be overcome through a computer link.

The promotion for the Pulse system would initially be through word of mouth and personal selling by the hospital marketing departments to selected physicians. The hospital director of Marketing, armed with a fact sheet and an agreement form, would call on physicians and office managers to present the concept, the product, and the procedures. Follow-up meetings would be conducted either by marketing representatives or staff of the Pulse system.

It was not anticipated that there would be obstacles to obtaining commitments from physicians to test the Pulse system in their offices. The greatest difficulty in selling the Pulse system was expected to be ensuring that ongoing support and service were consistently excellent. Customer satisfaction would determine the degree of acceptance of the Pulse system.

After installation had been completed, and the system was operating smoothly, the staff would continue to make periodic office visits at times convenient for office personnel. The purpose of the visits would be to reinforce previous training and demonstrate more sophisticated features of the system as they became available. At approximately four to six weeks after initial installation, marketing personnel would begin to monitor satisfaction and acceptance. Any concerns would be relayed to Information Services for immediate resolution. User satisfaction would be monitored by an annual survey.

In the long run, marketing of the Pulse system would depend on the response of the users. Physicians were believed to rely heavily on word of mouth for information regarding hospital projects. No amount of glib promotion by Samaritan would undo any bad press that might be generated by unhappy customers. After the product was deemed successful, SHS would develop a more formal or traditional product marketing communications plan.

The computer link would also be used in negotiations with HMOs, PPOs, and self-insured employers at the discretion of the SHS Contract Negotiating Team, headed by Regulatory Programs.

Relationship to Other Strategies

The Pulse system would be only one component of SHS's plan for developing closer relationships with physicians. Other elements included joint ventures, Samaritan Health Plan (an IPA HMO), a future discount on malpractice insurance for physicians who provided a high percentage of their admissions, and the future development of two or more multispecialty group practices, where 50–60 physicians would work for SHS on salary.

SHS management believed that the support of ambulatory care would be the important opportunity offered by physician-to-hospital links. The timeliness of data could be increased, leading to improved patient care outcomes. The Pulse system would link the proposed SHS group practice centers to SHS hospitals and other SHS businesses. The link would also support Samaritan Health Plan physicians by providing verification of coverage (and allow the plan to keep track of incurred expenses).

SHS management wanted to integrate the link into its physicians relations program. They did not view the link as a separate, distinct service. To implement this idea, SHS placed the marketing directors of each of its hospitals in charge of targeting the physicians to be offered the link, making the initial contact to explain the link, and providing feedback to the program staff in Information Services on physician satisfaction, desired improvements, and problems.

Current Procedures and Functions

Functions

As of April 1989, the Pulse system allowed the user to perform a number of functions:

1. *Select a Physician:* Selects the physician or group of physicians. Information would then be displayed only for the patients of that physician or group.

2. *Inpatient Census:* Displays inpatient census of selected physician(s), showing name, unit, room/bed, birth date, and hospital account number.

3. *All Patient List:* Displays an alphabetical list of all the patients in the system associated with the physician(s). After a name (or names) was selected, the type of patient (for example, inpatient, emergency room), sex, ethnic group/race, and birth date would be shown. A specific patient could be listed by entering the patient's last name.

4. *Recent Patients:* Displays an alphabetical list of all patients in the system whose last names match the name entered into the system. After a name was selected, the type of patient (for example, inpatient, emergency room), sex, ethnic group/race, and birth date would be shown.

5. *Patient Names and Histories:* Displays an alphabetical list of all patients in the system whose last names match the name entered into the system. After a name was selected, information on the ten most recent visits to the hospital would be displayed.

The following functions could be performed after a patient name had been selected. A warning would be displayed if the physician selected from the master screen was not involved in the care of the patient. The names of the physicians displayed would depend on the user's identification number and password.

6. *Demographic Information:* Displays demographic data on patients selected.

7. *Insurance Information:* Displays information needed to bill a third party.

8. *Lab Results Inquiry:* Provides on-line access to most laboratory test results except dictated pathology and x-ray reports.

9. *Medical Record Abstract:* Provides a summary of the admission, and the diagnosis and procedure codes.

10. *ED Log Inquiry:* Provides summary information on a patient's visit to the emergency room.

11. *Display Orders:* Provides a listing of clinical and supply orders entered into the system.

SHS hospitals have not been interested in preadmission or order entry. The hospitals believed that data entered by a physician's office would be less accurate than data entered by hospital personnel. Order entry was not desired because nurses on the floor would be bypassed, and they were required to confirm telephone orders. Since they must speak with the physician anyway, the hospitals believed time would not be saved.

Physicians could not communicate with each other without going through the central computer at SHS. SHS management wanted to make the hospital the core of the system. Management also believed that physicians would always view the system as controlled by the hospital, even if the host computer was not the hospital's main computer. Physicians who were reluctant to join the system because they did not want the hospital to have access to their data would still view the computer as controlled by the hospital, even if it was owned by a separate corporation.

Use of Terminal Emulation

SHS decided not to write its own PC-based user interface, but to distribute terminal emulation software to physicians. This was done for a number of reasons. SHS did not want to write PC software and support various operating systems. Terminal emulation meant that the link would use the same programming language and operating system as SHS's main computer.

The major disadvantage was that physicians could not insert data obtained from the link directly into billing forms and other records. Data had to be converted to an appropriate file format, downloaded as a file, and then inserted where needed. SHS found during the pilot that physician office staff printed out the data they needed and reentered the data into their own computer systems. However, most physicians had only a few patients in the hospital, so reentering the data was not very time consuming. SHS believed that the work involved in writing software that would insert data directly into a physician's office records was not justified.

The use of terminal emulation means that the user must understand various system messages. To assist the user, SHS distributed a user's guide. Users might receive the messages shown in Table 12.3, indicating that they should not enter messages, when connected to the host computer using a PC and modem. The use of symbols and messages, rather than statements in English, could present a problem for those who only use PC software. Although a regular user of the Pulse system would not have a problem, an occasional user could find the messages a deterrent to use of the system.

On the other hand, SHS avoided the expense of writing a program that would translate its system messages into terms closer to spoken English (i.e., a special user interface). SHS encouraged the vendors of practice management software to do this job for the physicians' they served. If SHS had written a user interface itself, it still would not have been identical to the one being used by physicians who purchased practice management, word-processing, or other PC software.

Assistance for Users

SHS staff spent about 45 minutes per office training staff in the use of the Pulse system. In addition, the Network Control Center for the Pulse system,

Table 12.3   Pulse System Messages

PC-System	Meaning
X []	Terminal wait. Time is required for the host system to perform a function. Wait.
X ? +	What? The last operation was not accepted. Check to make sure the operation you want to perform is correct. Then press RESET and try again.
X SYSTEM	System lock. The host system has locked your keyboard. Look for a message. Wait or press RESET.

within the Information Services Department of SHS, had a help desk that was staffed 24 hours a day, 7 days a week to assist in analyzing application software and hardware problems.

Pulse contained a number of features to help the user. The bottom of each screen contains a HELP command that could be selected. A description of the screen function would then be displayed. By selecting MODEL, the user could see an example of a completed screen.

The first screen that a user saw after signing on (i.e., connecting to Pulse) allowed the user to begin a tutorial, to read a description of support services available and obtain the telephone number for support, and to look up the most commonly used telephone numbers at the user's Samaritan hospital.

Security

SHS used a dial-back system to ensure that a call was coming from an authorized telephone. When a call was received, the SHS mainframe hung up and dialed back the authorized telephone number for the user involved (for example, the physician's office).

Each user was given both an individual identification number (ID) and a password. The system used these to determine the access level, that is, what data the user was allowed to see and the functions the user might perform. Pulse used terminal emulation, so that the user was linking to SHS's Samaritan Patient Information Network (SPIN), which included most patient data held in the computer.

When the user signed on, a list of physician names was displayed that corresponded to the user's password and ID. For example, physicians would see their names and the names of physicians in their group, if any. Physician office staff would see the names of the physicians they worked with.

If the user sought information (other than name) for a patient who was not being treated by a physician on their list, a warning screen appeared. If the user continued the request, the information would be displayed, but the system would audit the activity, and justification might be required.

Access would only be denied if the patient had specifically requested that no information be released as a condition of admission. In this case, only physicians associated with the case would be able to access data.

This was SHS's solution to the problem of determining who has a legitimate right to information on a patient. The hospital might have sought to keep track of all consultations requested, the physicians who have been asked to cover for an absent physician, and other reasons why a physician not directly involved with a patient's care might seek information on a patient. Because of the complexity of this process, and the possibility that information might be denied to a physician who needed it, SHS chose to simply record who asked for and obtained access to patient information to allow further investigation.

A physician could be added to a patient's record by notifying Patient Services at the specific hospital or by asking nursing to enter an order for a consult.

Evaluation

Evaluation Plan

The business plan for the Pulse system outlined a plan for evaluation. Included in the evaluation would be the following components:

1. Installation profile and analysis of the practice including:
   — number of physicians
   — admitting pattern (past 12 months)
   — number of years in practice
   — use of the system
   — inpatient utilization statistics (charges, length of stay by diagnosis-related group) after implementation
   — outpatient utilization statistics that have been effected through the network
   — level of automation
   — type of specialists
   — HMO affiliation
   — results of surveys (6, 12, and 24 months after implementation)
2. Cost to provide the service:
   — personnel
   — system utilization
3. Impact on SHS operations:
   — increased efficiency estimated by affected departments

— perception of administrators of improved communications with physicians

— offset costs, such as mail

To determine the success of the system, linked physicians would be compared with nonlinked control groups to see if practice patterns change following installation. The three control groups would include:

— physicians from the same specialty and size of practice

— physicians with stable practices (no retirements, deaths, or major effects from HMOs)

— physicians with loyalties to SHS similar to those of physicians in the linked group

SHS would acquire a computer tape from the Arizona state health department that included the license numbers of physicians involved in treating hospital inpatients. Using its own list of physician license numbers, SHS would determine where its physicians were admitting and treating patients. The data tape was available every six months for about $35. This would allow SHS to determine if physicians using the link changed their patterns of admission to various hospitals. An additional admission was worth an average of $1,700 to SHS.

SHS management calculated the revenues, expenses, and case flow required under a number of scenarios (for example, no additional admissions per installation per year, and two additional admissions). SHS estimated that if half of the installations had existing hardware and the other half required hardware, and each installation generated two more admissions per year, the Pulse system would be profitable in the second year of operation (see Exhibit 12.1).

SHS management expected there were three other ways that the investment in the Pulse system could be recouped. First, there was evidence that SHS could increase utilization of some outpatient services if it was able to process patients and deliver results competitively. Second, physicians might be able to discharge patients more quickly if they received diagnostic test results on a timely basis. Third, the Pulse system might help physicians to make more efficient use of their time, which would induce them to refer additional patients to SHS facilities when possible.

Results

As of early 1989, SHS had not determined if there was a change in the number of admissions of physicians who used the link.

The SHS computer periodically produced a report that showed the number of transactions by type (for example, lab results inquiry) for each site. Also produced is a report that shows the number of transactions, by type of transaction. This allowed management to determine, for example, how many times a site requested insurance information compared to other sites on the system.

Growth of the Link

The SHS began marketing the Pulse system in November 1988. By March 1989, 16 groups with 56 physicians were on-line, as well as an HMO with 40 physicians. The groups ranged in size from one to ten physicians. All the sites were in the Phoenix metropolitan area.

As of March 1989, there was no discernible pattern in terms of the age, size, or specialty of the groups signing contracts. Groups did, however, predominate. Older physicians were signing on to use the Pulse system.

One vendor had developed the software to link to SHS's computer. SHS had begun to receive calls from this vendor's customers, who wanted to begin communications with SHS.

Growth in the number of sites had, however, been slower than expected. There are several possible explanations. Marketing of the system was initially by informal communications, and by formal presentations by the hospital marketing directors. In January 1989, Pulse staff took over the marketing effort, partly because of the departure of hospital marketing staff. In six weeks, there were 13 additional contracts signed. SHS management believed that the slow growth during the first three months was because hospital marketing directors did not have the time to call physicians and make presentations. When they did make a presentation, the marketing staff, who lacked technical knowledge, could not provide solutions to hardware and software problems, or provide estimated prices.

The SHS manager in charge of the Pulse system interviewed physician office staff over the telephone, determined what hardware and software were needed, mailed a price quote, and then followed up with a telephone call. Demonstrations, where the staff person who had to carry out a task (for example, retrieve billing information) could be shown how easy it was, were also quickly scheduled. SHS staff could also provide solutions to hardware and software problems at the demonstrations.

SHS management believed that the difference between using Information Systems (IS), as opposed to marketing, staff was the speed with which technical problems could be solved and prices quoted. SHS management felt that these were the major obstacles for some physician offices, and IS staff could solve them faster because of their technical knowledge.

The problem of coordinating the marketing of the Pulse system with other efforts to market to physicians was solved by having Pulse staff call physicians from a priority list developed by individual SHS hospitals. Pulse staff called the administrators in charge of physician relations and told them who would be called. The administrators could then provide comments and suggestions, and ask Pulse staff to drop some names from the list or postpone the call.

The decision to have physicians purchase their own hardware may also have been responsible for the slow growth in the number of physicians participating. Some physicians were very price-sensitive. Some had complained that they could get better prices on hardware by purchasing from discounters (who offered no support). Others had refused to purchase relatively inexpensive hardware needed to use their existing computers, including a $50 A/B switch that would allow one line of an office PBX (private branch exchange) telephone system to be used for the link.

Pulse system staff believed they had greater success with physicians who needed to make smaller investments, with consulting physicians who needed data to bill for their services, and with physicians who had already decided to computerize but had not yet done so. One primary care physician was willing to pay $16 for the computer cable needed to install the link, but not several hundred dollars for a printer. A specialist who provided consultations was willing to pay several thousand dollars; the specialist did not have the data already collected by the attending physician's office staff and needed hospital data to bill.

Price sensitivity might be related to the benefits of the link as perceived by the physicians. A survey undertaken to evaluate the pilot showed that:

— physicians were interested in accessing data from the hospital computer but were less sure whether networking between physicians was practical at that time.

— hospitals and physicians shared a desire to streamline the admitting process. However, physicians did not think that the computer would be able to save time.

When SHS asked the physicians at the 12 pilot sites to indicate the importance of existing and potential tasks that could be carried out over the link, none was rated as very important by a majority. These tasks included the retrieval of lab results and inpatient financial information for billing.

What explains the low rating given to retrieving important information quickly? One explanation was that not enough could be done over the link. When asked why retrieving lab results was not rated more highly, one physician responded that significant lab results usually meant that other tests needed to be ordered. The physician would then have to call the hospital anyway. Why not just make one call and get the results over the telephone?

Another explanation was that physicians were not retrieving the information before, and therefore did not value the new system. The benefits were being received by the physician's office staff.

The low ratings given by pilot study participants to the value of having access to SHS data suggested to management that simply increasing the type of data that physicians could access may not be enough to stimulate growth in the number of physicians acquiring the link.

Future Development

Enhancements

As of April 1989, SHS management was planning to add results reporting and the transmission of radiology images, and to allow physicians to look at the schedules of hospital services and other physicians. To increase the benefits of the link, SHS was considering giving physicians access to PROFS (IBM's Professional Office System), which includes electronic mail and a calendar. Physicians could then look at other physician's office schedules and make a request for an appointment for their patients. They could also exchange messages. PROFS could also be used to provide a channel of communication with management to solve physicians' problems, for example, parking, late lab tests, and questions about hospital procedures. SHS was, however, concerned that the electronic mail function would be used to bypass established channels for communication, producing conflict.

The Health Care Financing Administration issued regulations in late 1988 allowing physicians, in lieu of a signature, to use a physician-specific alphanumeric code to attest to the accuracy of the principal and secondary diagnoses and the major procedures performed, a necessary step before an inpatient bill can be submitted for a Medicare beneficiary. A biometric system that could identify physicians by reading their fingerprints could also be used.

This opened up the possibility of using the link to solve the problem of getting physicians to do the attestation quickly and could potentially save SHS money, since the submission of a bill had to be delayed until these signatures were obtained. Using the link would allow office staff to monitor the records that physicians must review and help the hospital and physician obtain a timely review. Physicians would also be able to review the information while in their offices at their convenience, rather than only on visits to the hospital.

On the horizon were other opportunities. SHS could offer electronic claims processing to groups through vendors such as Oakmark and Cross Shield of Arizona, which would enable SHS to penetrate the market more quickly.

Management did not believe that it was to SHS's advantage to offer reference data on drugs, treatment, and procedures through the Pulse system since this information was already available through a subsidiary of the American Medical Association (AMA). American Medical Computing had begun marketing AMA/Net to area physicians. AMA/Net offered access to medical data bases and information from sources such as Medline, the National Library of Medicine's data base of abstracts from medical journals. SHS did not want to compete with the AMA, nor did SHS feel it had a more valuable product to offer. Offering this service would also not differentiate SHS from its competitors.

SHS management felt that the highest priority should be given to providing certification of benefits and tracking incurred, but not reported, services for physicians participating in SHS's IPA HMO. This would provide a tangible benefit for physicians and SHS.

Management also believed that a payoff for SHS would come from using the link as an enhancement of services offered to employers. SHS wanted to offer large employers access to data, especially notification of admissions and charges incurred. This would allow employers to implement their certification procedures for cost control more effectively.

Pace of Development

SHS had the advantage of having as competitors a hospital that failed in its first attempt at establishing a link and another that lacked the resources to develop one. Management believed that only the Mayo Clinic could move quickly to develop a link.

Mayo was effectively competing with SHS in the Phoenix area. SHS management believed that there were no enhancements to the Pulse system currently available that would offer SHS a competitive advantage over the Mayo Clinic. Management believed, however, that the scope and completeness of SHS's data bases provided SHS with a major resource.

Management believed that SHS had the opportunity to develop a low-cost link slowly, adding services as they were requested by physicians and where they appeared valuable to SHS. The end result would be a system that contained many small features that collectively were highly valued by physicians. This might allow the hospital to achieve part of the competitive advantage that might have resulted from the more expensive strategy of distributing free hardware and software, including a practice management system.

The slow growth in the numbers of physicians signing up for Pulse had not resulted in any thought about abandoning the link. SHS management saw it as a low-cost, long-term strategy for improving physician relationships. SHS management believed the link was essential for holding and maintaining the loyalty of physicians.

13.

Vassar Brothers Hospital's Development of a Hospital-to-Physician Computer Link

Introduction

Vassar Brothers Hospital is a 300-bed hospital located in Poughkeepsie, New York. In August 1988, it began a pilot project that linked three medical groups and one solo physician to the hospital's computers.

The objective of the hospital was to begin learning about the needs and desires of physicians and the technical requirements of a computer link. If the pilot developed into a regular service to physicians, the hospital hoped it would increase physician loyalty and result in increased inpatient admissions and the use of outpatient services.

Market Area and Competitive Environment

Competitors

Two hospitals are located in Poughkeepsie, New York, a city of about 70,000 people that is 1½ hours drive north of New York City. While Vassar Brothers

This case was prepared by Roger Kropf, Ph.D., for publication and use in classroom discussion, rather than to illustrate either effective or ineffective handling of an administrative situation. The author wishes to thank the following Vassar Brothers Hospital managers for their generous support in the preparation of this case: Richard Colesanti, Director of Management Information Systems; Thomas A. Dee, Vice-President, Professional/Support Services; Charles M. Gill, Vice-President, Corporate Development; and Duncan Chisholm, Programmer/Analyst.

Hospital and St. Francis Hospital (a 295-bed Catholic hospital) compete for physicians and patients, the two hospitals have also cooperated. The two hospitals have agreed that Vassar Brothers Hospital will provide an array of specialized services, such as radiation oncology. St. Francis has focused its attention on mental health and alcohol and drug abuse services, in addition to providing a range of primary acute care services. Neither hospital is affiliated with a medical school. However, St. Francis Hospital is expected to begin a family practice residency program in 1990.

The two hospitals do compete, however. Both hospitals applied for a certificate of need for a cardiac catheterization lab in 1987. Both hospitals started a physician referral service. Both have an "eldercare" program that offers special services to older residents who join.

Vassar Brothers Hospital's senior management believes that the two hospitals will continue to compete for some services and cooperate in providing others. New York State Department of Health guidelines and regulations make it important to demonstrate cooperative planning, especially for expensive specialized services.

Vassar Brothers Hospital had approximately an 80 percent average occupancy in 1988. Even though occupancy is high, hospital management is still concerned about inpatient market share and the growing market for outpatient services. Strict regulation of hospital rates by the State Department of Health and the U.S. Department of Health and Human Services severely limits the profitability of inpatient services and makes it important for the hospital to monitor its current volume of patients.

Physicians

Hospital management felt that Poughkeepsie was a place where many physicians aligned themselves with one of the hospitals, becoming a "Vassar doctor" or "St. Francis doctor." However, many physicians divide their admissions between Vassar Brothers Hospital and St. Francis Hospital. Eighty percent of the physicians had admitting privileges at both hospitals. The hospitals will continue to compete for physicians, and physicians are interested in support from local hospitals for a number of reasons.

HMO market share has grown, and the largest HMO, HealthShield, is a staff-model HMO that is owned by an HMO in the Albany, New York, area. Like other attractive areas close to both rural farmland and large cities, Poughkeepsie has also seen an increase in new physicians entering the area. The area had the lowest unemployment rate in New York State in 1988, the result of new jobs from established employers like IBM and a growing number of high-tech industries entering the area.

To serve physicians better, Vassar Brothers Hospital began a group purchasing program that offered lower prices on supplies to member physicians, a newsletter for physicians, the computer link, and a physician referral service.

A 24-hour physician hot line was introduced that physicians could use to ask questions and make complaints. A voice messaging system was installed that would allow physicians to leave a message when they got no answer. Radiologists could also use the system to dictate test results.

The computer link was another strategy to improve services and overcome the effects of tight staffing, which sometimes resulted in telephones not being answered promptly. Management was aware that Vassar Brothers Hospital had the reputation among physicians of being a place where it was harder to get things done. They believed that this was true, and partly the result of tighter staffing patterns. While Vassar Brothers Hospital's FTE staff per bed was 2.8 in 1988, St. Francis had 4.1 FTE staff per bed. Management wanted to introduce technology to improve services to physicians and avoid having to increase staff in a tight labor market. The use of telecommunications and computer technology was also consistent with the hospital's attempt to position itself as the hospital that offered the latest technology to the community.

Development of a Computer Link

Staffing

Vassar Brothers Hospital developed the link by taking a number of actions. A programmer/analyst (who had previously been a respiratory therapist at the hospital) was assigned as installation manager for the link. He worked on the necessary programming and hardware and software acquisition, trained the office staff of physicians, troubleshot, and periodically visited the offices. He was also given a variety of other jobs in data processing as the need arose but kept microcomputers as the focus of his work.

Vendor Selection

The hospital acquired DOCNET from Compucare (an information systems vendor in Virginia) for $15,000. The Vassar Brothers Hospital computer system had been directly managed by Compucare until early 1985, and the hospital's major pieces of software were written by Compucare. No outside vendor or consultant was used to develop the link. The hospital did, however, add many new features to DOCNET.

Hardware and Software Costs

Vassar Brothers Hospital budgeted $75,000 for hardware and software for the link. This included $15,000 for the DOCNET software license and $22,000 for hardware (3 used PCs and 4 modems, 16 additional ports for the Data General minicomputer and 16 modems for the ports). The remaining funds were to be spent as needed on hardware for the hospital's Data General computer to handle additional sites and transactions performed.

Pilot Participant Selection

Vassar Brothers Hospital called its system DocLink. One solo practice and three physician groups were linked to the hospital's computers. One group had 3 physicians, and the other two had 8 and 17 physicians. The solo practitioner was chosen because he was an interested and capable microcomputer user. The two larger groups were chosen because their physicians admitted patients only to Vassar Brothers, and they were the two largest groups on the medical staff. The solo physician and three-person group split their admissions between Vassar Brothers Hospital and St. Francis.

Use of Terminal Emulation

Physicians' offices were provided with communications software that automatically dialed a telephone number and connected their computer with a Data General minicomputer at Vassar Brothers Hospital. Once the office was connected to the hospital's computer, the user saw a menu of the functions available. Once they had selected a function, the user saw the same screens and used the same commands as anyone else in the hospital. There was no special user interface (i.e., a special set of menus, graphics, or commands) other than the initial DocLink menu.

Functions Performed

The DOCNET software given to the four pilot sites included the following functions:

1. *Patient List:* Retrieve/print a list of inpatients and their room numbers for an individual physician.
2. *Group Patient List:* Retrieve/print a list of inpatients and their room numbers for all physicians in a group.
3. *Patient Inquiry:* Retrieve/print demographic information on patients.
4. *Physicians in House:* Sign in and out of the hospital, and look at which physicians are in the hospital and in surgery.

5. *Incomplete Charts:* Retrieve/print a list of the charts not completed by a physician.

6. *Clinical Data:* Retrieve/print lab test results, radiology result transcriptions, history and physicals, and any other transcriptions in the medical record.

7. *Message:* Send, delete, redisplay, or review messages.

8. *Consult:* Request a consultation for an inpatient.

Expected Benefits for Physicians

The link offered a number of benefits to physicians:

— Their staff could retrieve information faster by bypassing the telephone system.

— The information was more accurate because it was not spoken over the telephone, written down, and then typed.

— Physicians could locate their patients in the hospital quickly.

— Office staff could determine that the physician had been asked to provide a consult and could then initiate the necessary billing when completed. Some physicians neglected to tell staff when they provided a consult or to provide the information for billing.

Although DocLink could be modified to allow physician-to-physician communication, this was not a feature offered to the pilot sites. Physicians could communicate to each other through the hospital's computer using the message function.

Evaluation

The use of the system could be measured by the computer, which recorded whose password and identification number was used to carry out each inquiry and what data were retrieved. The office manager in each physician's office assigned identification codes to individual users, and their use of the system could be tracked.

One potential problem in measurement was that the link might be established with one password and identification number and then used by different people during the day. Vassar Brothers Hospital installed a program that checked once a minute to see if a transaction was being performed, and broke the link if one was not. This was for security reasons, but also allowed the system to more accurately record who was using the system.

Based on five months of data, the only physician who personally used the computer was the physician in solo practice. Use in three of the offices grew, while in one office no use was made of the link.

The office manager in that 17-physician group requested that the computer be put in the business office at the other end of the building from where patient care was provided. She also did not issue codes to nurses. When asked, several physicians in this group stated that they did not know the link existed and had been asking their nurses to call the hospital for information.

Vassar Brothers Hospital hoped in the future to compare the number of transactions performed by physicians' offices to the number of their inpatient admissions. Since two of the four sites (with 25 of the 29 physicians on the link) admitted their inpatients exclusively to Vassar Brothers, this evaluation has not been a high priority. The hospital also collected data on the number of outpatient service referrals by each physician, so it could determine if they were increasing.

Future Development

At the end of five months, hospital management agreed that expansion of the system was desirable, but a number of decisions had to be made:

— Who would pay the cost of hardware in physicians' offices?
— Should loyal physicians, those who split admissions, or nonusers be given priority?
— What type of person should be hired to increase staff for this function?
— What else should physicians be allowed to do over the link?
— What method should be used to evaluate the effectiveness of the system?

Three of the four offices in the pilot phase had been given a PC and a modem on loan, and the fourth office had been lent two modems to use with their own PCs. The hospital felt it could not afford to distribute free equipment to other offices. The question was what to charge physicians. The hospital was willing to pay its own hardware costs. It planned to install 16 modems and additional ports to the Data General minicomputer, and would purchase further hardware if necessary.

The question was how much to charge physicians, and how many physicians would buy the necessary equipment. The hospital was also considering offering practice management services through an affiliation agreement with a consulting firm. This would partly solve the hardware price issue since physicians would buy their hardware as part of a practice management package. A major concern, however, was finding a consulting firm or vendor who would provide high quality services and products since the hospital's reputation with physicians was at risk. The hospital decided to proceed slowly in developing such an alliance.

Another potential problem was the reluctance of physicians to allow hospital staff to see their data. Several physicians had already expressed concern that the hospital would be able to look at their billing data using the existing link. Although it was explained to them that this was technically impossible, they were not completely convinced. The implementation of a practice management system that included billing, accounts receivable, and a general ledger package would require that a vendor or hospital staff gain access to, or create, computer data bases of financial data. Some physicians might not purchase a practice management system from the hospital or an affiliated vendor for this reason.

If the physicians were offered any kind of subsidy, the selection of physicians would be a major problem. The hospital could offer the subsidized hardware to loyal physicians (who admitted patients only to Vassar Brothers Hospital) but then would not realize increases in revenue. If it offered the subsidized system to physicians who split their referrals, it would anger the exclusive admitters but might gain referrals and revenue. The hospital had to make a difficult choice.

The programmer/analyst in charge of the link was becoming a valued systems professional. Some of the work involved in expanding the system clearly did not require his level of expertise (for example, training new office staff). A less expensive professional was needed, one with some computer expertise, good communication skills, and knowledge of (or at least the ability to sensitively handle) the problems of physician office management.

It was not clear where such a person would come from, how many were needed, and what they should be paid. The Information Systems Department hired programmers with associate degrees and trained them. This was one option, but clearly the skills needed were different. The director of Management Information Systems also felt he lacked norms for the hiring of this type of professional, including norms for how much time it should take to install hardware, train staff, and perform the other tasks required to incorporate a physician's office into the system, and what salary to pay.

The hospital intended to enhance the system by including outpatient service scheduling, and pharmacy and dietary ordering. In the original system, physicians could view what lab and radiology services had been ordered but could not order services. Vassar Brothers Hospital felt that physicians ordering services on the system would bypass the nurses, who would have to call the physicians anyway to confirm the order. The hospital preferred that physicians order services while at the hospital, or through a telephone call to a nurse.

Because of the loyalties of physicians, Vassar Brothers Hospital management believed that the link was more likely to affect the use of outpatient, rather than inpatient, services. They believed that 80 percent of all outpatient services were scheduled by the physician's office, so efforts to increase the use of Vassar Brothers Hospital should focus on the physician, rather than consumers. The scheduling of outpatient services was the next service that Vassar Brothers Hospital wanted to offer over the computer link.

The hospital intended to develop a file transfer protocol that would allow the transfer of files to a microcomputer in a standard format called ASCII (American Standard Code for Information Interchange). The physician's office staff might then be able to enter the data into their own systems, for example, for billing. Discussions were held with office managers to assist them in doing this, since it would make it unnecessary for their staff to reenter data.

As of early 1989, Vassar Brothers Hospital management believed that it was a real possibility that St. Francis Hospital would also develop a link. A task force was convened at Vassar Brothers to decide on the rate of growth and future direction of the physician-to-hospital computer link.

14.

Inter+Net Health System's Implementation of a Health Information and Referral Service

Introduction

Inter+Net Health System was formed by 13 not-for-profit hospitals in the Washington, D.C., area in 1987. It was formed to take advantage of economies of scale and permit its members to offer a network of providers to employers and other payers who wanted to contract for services. The members of Inter+Net were initially interested in starting a PPO to compete in the Washington area. They were also interested in other activities that would help them develop a cohesive regional health system. A telemarketing and service referral program was one such activity.

In October 1988, Inter+Net began operating an Ask-A-Nurse® health information and referral service for the Washington, D.C., area (Ask-A-Nurse is a registered trademark of Referral Systems Group, Inc., Citrus

This case was prepared by Roger Kropf, Ph.D, for publication and use in classroom discussion, rather than to illustrate either effective or ineffective handling of an administrative situation. The author wishes to thank the following Inter+Net Health System managers for their generous support in the preparation of this case: Donald R. Wallace, President; Marshall de G. Ruffin, Jr., M.D., Senior Vice-President; Nancy Schamber, Ask-A-Nurse Product Manager; Mary Dockham, R.N., Ask-A-Nurse Nursing Manager; Jerilyn Woelfel, Ask-A-Nurse Systems Manager; and Mona Johnston, Ask-A-Nurse Director of Marketing.

Heights, California). Ask-A-Nurse was a program offered by the Referral Systems Group, which sold exclusive licenses to use the program in a specific market. Referral Systems Group provided the necessary computer software, training, marketing materials, and technical support to implement and maintain the program.

Ask-A-Nurse put a registered nurse wearing a telephone headset in front of a computer terminal. Incoming calls were channeled to the nurse, who spoke to callers while entering data into the terminal. There was no charge to the caller. The nurse asked for the caller's name, address, and other information, which were stored in a central data base. Information on physicians and other services in the community that would be helpful to the caller could be retrieved. Other information (for example, a symptom or problem) was used to retrieve medical protocols that helped the nurse assess the caller's problem.

This case describes the environment faced by Inter+Net managers and the strategies they developed; the selection, marketing, and implementation of the Ask-A-Nurse system; the technical procedures and functions of the system; evaluation procedures and results; the status of the Ask-A-Nurse system as of early 1989; and management's plans for future development.

Market Area and Competitive Environment

The Washington, D.C., metropolitan area has 3.5 million residents served by 39 hospitals. Hospitals operating within the District of Columbia face very different conditions from those in the surrounding suburbs in Maryland and Virginia.

District of Columbia

Although the District of Columbia had the second-highest per capita income, 21 percent of the population lacked health insurance, and 14 percent lived in poverty. Population declined 1 percent from 1980–86, falling to 638,000.[1] The District of Columbia had the sixth-largest number of AIDS cases among metropolitan areas in 1988; the U.S. Centers for Disease Control reported a total of 2,220 cases as of October 31, 1988.[2] Drug-related health problems and deaths had also increased. Drug-related emergency department cases rose from 4,213 in 1984 to 6,285 in 1986.[3] At 494-bed Greater Southeast Community Hospital (an Inter+Net Health System member), 40 percent of the women who delivered babies there were substance abusers.[4]

In 1987, hospitals in the district reported a total of $160 million in charity care and bad debt.[5] The expense of caring for the uninsured helped push costs at district hospitals to the fourth highest in the nation, $664 per day in 1986.[6] District hospitals needed to attract suburban patients, who are generally better insured, but the proportion of suburban patients in district hospitals fell from 49 percent in 1982 to 42 percent in 1985.

Suburban Washington

Surrounding suburban areas in Maryland and Virginia were growing in population, and a higher proportion of their residents were insured. Suburban hospitals were offering more tertiary services and were keeping a growing share of suburban patients, often at lower cost. Kaiser Foundation Health Plan, one of three HMOs in Washington, did not contract with any district hospitals, in part because their costs were so much higher.[7]

Competitors

Medlantic, the only hospital system in the District of Columbia, operated four facilities with a total of 1,728 beds. It also had affiliate agreements with five hospitals outside the district that paid fees in exchange for management consulting, access to clinical programs, and discounts on services. In addition, the system's for-profit division, Medlantic Enterprises, operated 14 health care facilities and related businesses.[8] Medlantic had spent considerable money creating public awareness of the Medlantic name. It had developed a referral service for all its facilities and services.

The two dominant HMOs in the Washington, D.C., area were Kaiser (a group model) and Group Health (a staff model). There were also several IPAs, which Inter+Net management felt had alienated physicians in the area. Inter+Net Health System, therefore, did not face competition from a large, dominant HMO or PPO.

Employers

Inter+Net management felt that employers were a major market for Inter+Net because employers wanted high-quality, cost-effective services. To achieve that objective, employers needed and wanted:

— a cohesive network for providing care that could prove it offered coordinated, high-quality services, and that could handle administrative tasks such as claims processing and utilization review

— help in informing their employees of the benefits they were eligible for and where they could get services

— help in influencing employees to manage their medical problems appropriately and reduce the indiscriminate use of medical services

Physicians

Physicians in the suburban areas were busy and did not feel intense pressure to join alternative delivery systems and accept discounts. Inter+Net believed it was important that its members educated physicians on such systems and provided them with experience in evaluating contracts offered by PPOs, HMOs, third-party payers, and employers.

Strategy Development

Management believed that Inter+Net's primary focus should be on payers, especially self-insured employers. Inter+Net's primary strategy was to develop a regional health system without requiring member hospitals and their physicians to merge into a single corporate entity. With one-third of all hospital beds and thousands of physicians spread over the metropolitan area, they believed that Inter+Net would be very attractive to payers if its members and physicians could deliver services in a coordinated way.

There were a number of reasons for this strategy:

— To compete effectively, they believed Inter+Net had to convince employers and other third-party payers that it was an entity capable of organizing, managing, and delivering care across a large metropolitan area.

— To avoid having administrative structures (such as utilization review, membership services, referral systems, and quality assurance programs) imposed on its members by payers, Inter+Net should act like a regional health system and develop the administrative structures itself and sell them to payers.

— Inter+Net members were not interested in a merger of assets, and member hospitals and physicians wanted to choose which contracts they would enter into.

Inter+Net management hoped that in five years people in the Washington, D.C., area would say that they get their care from Inter+Net Health System, and mean by that an identifiable, cohesive network of providers with a great reputation for high-quality care and convenient, accessible service. The two major tools for creating coordination and cohesion would be the contracts Inter+Net would sign with payers and the information services that Inter+Net could provide. In order to understand the rationale for this strategy and the steps taken to implement it, some understanding of Inter+Net Health System and its members is required.

Background Information on Inter+Net Health System

Inter+Net Health System was a voluntary association of 13 hospitals that utilized thousands of physicians and hundreds of outpatient facilities to provide care to a metropolitan area. Exhibit 14.1 shows the locations of Inter+Net Health System hospitals. Inter+Net hospitals had a total of 3,591 licensed beds in 1988. In 1986, Inter+Net Health System hospitals had 33 percent of the discharges in the Washington, D.C., metropolitan area. Total net patient revenues were $637 million. The average occupancy of Inter+Net hospitals was 77 percent (versus 75 percent for other hospitals in the metro area). Occupancy rates ranged from 57 to 92 percent.

The hospitals in Inter+Net varied tremendously in size, from 131-bed Physicians Memorial Hospital in La Plata, Maryland, to 656-bed Fairfax Hospital in Falls Church, Virginia. Its members included both university teaching facilities, such as 539-bed Georgetown University Hospital in Washington, and community hospitals, like Frederick Memorial Hospital in rural Frederick County, Maryland. Four hospitals with 1,200 beds in the northern Virginia suburbs, including Fairfax Hospital, were owned by Fairfax Hospital System. Fairfax Hospital Systems' parent corporation was Inova Health Systems.

Member hospitals also owned four long-term care facilities with a total of 600 licensed beds. Seventeen ambulatory care centers were affiliated with Inter+Net Health System. Two of them were emergency care centers open 24 hours a day.

Services Provided to Members

Inter+Net Health System provided its members with a number of services:

— group negotiations of alternative delivery system contracts (for example, with a PPO or HMO)
— group purchasing arrangements
— clinical joint venture development
— administrative joint venture development
— lower interest rates for short- and long-term financing
— group marketing to consumers and employers

Alternative Delivery System Contracts

The physicians affiliated with Inter+Net Health System varied greatly in their willingness to enter into contracts. In the District of Columbia, Inter+Net had two established MeSh plans (an organization composed of the hospital

Exhibit 14.1   Map of Hospitals in Inter+Net Health System

 Inter+Net Health System

Suite 308, 1945 Old Gallows Road, Vienna, Virginia 22180 • 703-790-4669

HOSPITALS

Ⓐ Fairfax Hospital
Ⓑ Fair Oaks Hospital
Ⓒ Frederick Memorial Hospital
Ⓓ Georgetown University Hospital
Ⓔ Greater Southeast Community
Ⓕ Jefferson Hospital
Ⓖ Loudoun Hospital Center

Ⓗ Mount Vernon Hospital
Ⓘ Physicians Memorial Hospital
Ⓙ Potomac Hospital
Ⓚ Providence Hospital
Ⓛ Shady Grove Adventist Hospital
Ⓜ Washington Adventist Hospital

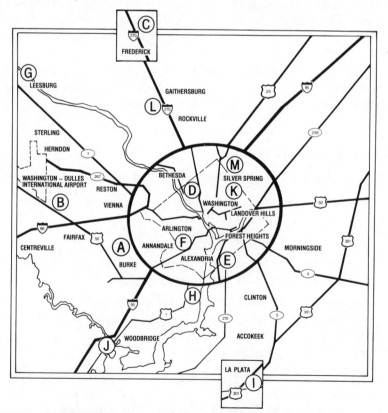

Source: Reprinted with the permission of Inter+Net Health System, Vienna, Virginia.

and physicians that engages in joint ventures), one at Providence and the other at Greater Southeast. They had five years of experience in contract negotiations with payers. They were ready to go when Inter+Net Health System started contracting.

At the other extreme, there were relatively few contracts in northern Virginia, where physicians were very busy. Physicians in northern Virginia started their own HMO to keep all other HMOs out—Physicians Health Plan/Physicians Care. It almost went bankrupt, and was acquired in late 1988 by Carefirst, an aggressive HMO from Baltimore. The physicians were reluctant to allow Inter+Net to organize them, fearing the growth of managed care systems in their areas.

Inter+Net Health System had met a lot of resistance from northern Virginia hospitals, who were busy. Even in northern Virginia, however, there were differences. Physicians affiliated with Potomac Hospital were threatened by a new Kaiser facility that was causing erosion in the number of paying patients.

One of the objectives in the formation of Inter+Net Health System was to develop a PPO that included member hospitals and affiliated physicians. That effort had moved slowly. Although Inter+Net had not decided whether to develop an PPO, it had decided to help its members deal cooperatively with the problem of deciding which PPOs and HMOs to join, and how to proceed with negotiations.

In 1988, Inter+Net organized a research effort financed by the joint ventures between member hospitals and their medical staffs (referred to as local provider units or LPUs). The LPUs contributed to the costs of hiring a consultant and legal team to research and produce detailed financial and operating profiles of HMOs, which was used in negotiations with the HMOs. The information included whether the HMO was frequently late in paying providers in other states, the number of days the insurer needed to pay a claim that had no mistakes, the type of risk pools that physicians were required to participate in, and what employers had contracts with the HMO.[9]

The development of this service was consistent with Inter+Net's strategy of attempting to demonstrate the benefits of cooperative action. In order to get hospitals and physicians to work together, management believed the knowledge and sophistication of both parties about contractual arrangements to provide services had to be increased. Providing information remained a key element in that strategy.

The next step in contracting would be to have Inter+Net negotiate contracts, which members and affiliated physicians could accept or reject. The result, however, would be a great need for readily available information (for both consumers and providers) on which hospitals and physicians were participating, what services were available, and how to obtain them.

Role of Information Services

Inter+Net management believed that various information services could play a major role in creating a cohesive health system and in carrying out the contracts that Inter+Net Health System would sign to provide services to self-insured employers and other payers. In a network like Inter+Net, physicians would belong to different HMOs and PPOs, and accept different insurance plans, unlike a group practice operated as a single corporate entity, where a decision on whether everyone would participate was made. This created a different need for information.

An information center was needed that provided a range of services. The center should link hospitals and physicians, and link them in such a way that physicians began referring to other physicians in the system, changing their referral patterns so that they were supporting other practitioners, creating what would evolve into a regional "super" group practice, not in a corporate sense, but in a marketing and referral sense.

The information center would be important because physicians would need to know who, among the physicians they knew, accepted the insurance the patient had. In the absence of an information center, it was the patient who would be asked to call member services for an HMO or PPO and find out which physicians could provide the services they needed. A sophisticated matching service was needed. Such a sophisticated matching service could be used to distinguish one network of providers from others affiliating with insurers.

These information services could also:

— create an identity for Inter+Net Health System apart from its members in the minds of the public and payers

— make Inter+Net Health System the point of first contact for consumers seeking answers to their questions about health topics and health services, increasing awareness of Inter+Net and providing easy access to the Inter+Net network of providers

— serve as the central information source and triage point (1) for consumers and payers for services offered by Inter+Net, possibly including a PPO or HMO, and (2) for self-insured employers, insurance companies, and other organizations that wanted to utilize Inter-+Net Health System to provide benefit and service information to consumers and providers

— provide the mechanism for collecting and analyzing data required by payers on services rendered, quality, and outcomes, replacing any system that might be imposed on Inter+Net and providing useful information for negotiations with payers

— allow for the efficient referral of patients within the Inter+Net Health System, even when providers were not personally known to each other

Coordination with Member Activities

These would not be easy objectives to achieve within a voluntary association. Member hospitals shared similar objectives. One group of hospitals in Inter-+Net Health System, for example, had spent approximately $2 million per year on their own physician referral system. A major question facing Inter-+Net was whether, and how, to integrate the efforts of its members that paralleled its own efforts.

The marketing directors of member hospitals had not always been supportive in discussions with Inter+Net about new efforts to develop and promote Inter+Net services. While their CEOs recognized the importance of a cohesive regional delivery system, their marketing directors perceived they were being evaluated by the results at an individual hospital. Other staff and physicians within member hospitals might feel the same way.

Selection of Ask-A-Nurse

One information service that was given a high priority was a physician referral service that would serve the Washington, D.C., area. Six member hospitals were already operating computer-based physician referral systems. A comprehensive report was prepared on the physician referral systems on the market in 1988. Ask-A-Nurse, a product of the Referral Systems Group of Citrus Heights, California, was finally selected for a number of reasons:

— It would provide health information as well as referrals and, there-fore, serve a wider range of needs and a larger number of consum-ers. Inter+Net would become a 24-hour-a-day, 7-day-a-week health information resource for the community.

— It would provide Inter+Net with an activity that would give high visibility and name recognition to Inter+Net, which was not well known.

— It would become operational quickly, since it utilized computer systems and procedures already in use in various metropolitan areas around the country.

— Inter+Net would be the first to offer this service in the Washington, D.C., area and an exclusive market-area license would prevent others from using the Ask-A-Nurse name and medical protocols.

Inter+Net believed that someone in the Washington area would otherwise get the license. Exclusivity also meant that an Inter+Net facility would lose the benefits of Ask-A-Nurse if they left Inter-+Net.

— It would provide measurable benefits to Inter+Net members in a short period of time in the form of additional hospital admissions, outpatient, and ER visits.

— It would allow member hospitals to provide a measurable benefit to their medical staffs in the form of additional patients.

Financial Feasibility Analysis

Tables 14.1 and 14.2 present the demand, revenue, and expense estimates made prior to the selection of Ask-A-Nurse. It was estimated that the Ask-A-Nurse system would produce revenues for member hospitals that exceeded costs by the end of one year, even without including the revenue that Inter-+Net physicians would receive as a result of increased referrals.

Based on experience at other Ask-A-Nurse sites, it was estimated that Inter+Net would receive 175,000 calls in a metropolitan area of 3.5 million in the first year. It was estimated that this would result in 10,500 ER visits and 980 hospital admissions.

Marginal hospital revenue resulting from the Ask-A-Nurse system was assumed to be 50 percent of the gross revenues. It was assumed that 50 percent would have been received anyway without the Ask-A-Nurse system. Marginal hospital costs for treating these patients was assumed to be 40 percent of marginal hospital revenue since Inter+Net Health System hospitals operated at less than capacity.

A sensitivity analysis of these two assumptions showed that the Ask-A-Nurse system became financially unattractive only if marginal hospital revenue was less than 35 percent (i.e., more than 65 percent of the revenues would have been received without the Ask-A-Nurse system) and marginal hospital cost was more than 40 percent of marginal revenue. Even then, the system would be attractive if the revenue to the physician was included. Marginal revenue was expected to exceed the sum of marginal costs and Ask-A-Nurse system operating costs by $378,991 the first year, that is, the Ask-A-Nurse system would be profitable.

Implementation and Marketing

Financing

The development of Ask-A-Nurse was funded by an assessment of each facility using a formula based on beds and gross revenue to determine how

Table 14.1 Ask-A-Nurse® Feasibility Study—Demand and Revenue Assumptions

Metro D.C. SMSA Population—3,500,000

Variables	Totals/Year
Estimated calls/year	175,000
ED referrals	38,500
ED visits	10,500
Inpatient admission from ED visits	560
Physician referrals	21,000
Inpatient admissions from physician referrals	420
Total admits from ED and MDs	980
Gross hospital revenues	
Gross revenue per ED visit	$1,312,500
Gross revenue per hospital admit	$4,900,000
Gross hospital revenue from Ask-A-Nurse referrals (does not include revenue from outpatient visits to hospital facilities, or other hospital services)	$6,212,500
Marginal hospital revenue from Ask-A-Nurse (revenue that is, on the margin, attributable to Ask-A-Nurse service)	$3,106,250
Marginal hospital costs (MHC) for hospital services provided	$1,242,500

Source: Excerpted from "An Analysis of a Health Information and Medical Services Matching Program for Inter+Net Health System," December 29, 1987. Reprinted with the permission of Referral Systems Group, Inc.

Table 14.2 Ask-A-Nurse® Feasibility Study—Projected Profitability in Year One

Revenues from Ask-A-Nurse	
Marginal hospital revenue from Ask-A-Nurse	$3,106,250
Marginal M.D. revenue from Ask-A-Nurse	$0
Total marginal revenue	$3,106,250
Marginal revenue per call	$17.75
Hospital marginal costs from Ask-A-Nurse referrals	$1,242,500
Operating costs of Ask-A-Nurse (Includes payroll, amortization of the start-up costs over 5 years, depreciation of capital equipment over 5 years, utilities, rent, supplies, support fees, and advertising)	$1,484,759
Total operating costs per call	$8.48
Marginal profit (Marginal revenue less marginal costs and operating costs)	$378,991
Total marginal profit per call	$2.17

Source: Excerpted from "An Analysis of a Health Information and Medical Services Matching Program for Inter+Net Health System," December 29, 1987. Reprinted with the permission of Referral Systems Group, Inc.

much each facility paid. Between September and December 1988, $1.4 million was invested in the acquisition of hardware and software, training, maintenance, and support, as well as salaries. The budget for 1989 was set at $1.5 million. Because of the size of the Washington area, Inter+Net expected demand to be high.

Staffing

When fully operational, Ask-A-Nurse was expected to have 25 FTE nurses, each a registered nurse (RN) with a minimum of two years experience. This included both a day and a night nurse manager. In addition, the system has a manager, a systems manager (responsible for technical support, including the hardware, and acting as liaison with the vendor), and a director of marketing. The nurse managers would devote 100 percent of their time to the system; the manager and systems manager would devote 80 percent of their time. The marketing director would be full-time. Ask-A-Nurse also had a medical director, who would spend 20 percent of his time working with the system.

Promotion

Because demand was expected to be high, only limited promotion of the Ask-A-Nurse system was undertaken during 1988. Inter+Net paid $116,000 for the inclusion of 19 ads in the *Washington Post* (see Exhibit 14.2) and $52,000 for 18 ads in the local newspapers. The ads ran between September 15 and November 31, 1988. Inter+Net Health System also paid $18,000 for 6 ads in the Washington-Baltimore *TV Guide*. Inter+Net's total print campaign for 1988 therefore cost about $186,000.

Inter+Net hired a public relations firm in 1988 to make contacts and increase the visibility of the Ask-A-Nurse system. The firm was paid approximately $100,000, and the equivalent of one staff member worked on Ask-A-Nurse over a three-month period. The firm helped place two public service announcements on television stations in the Washington area using text provided by the national vendor of the Ask-A-Nurse system. Ask-A-Nurse's medical director, manager, and staff also participated in dozens of interviews on the radio and television.

Inter+Net also volunteered to service the hot line for drug and alcohol information for a show entitled "City under Siege" that ran five nights a week for 13 weeks from 11:00–11:30 P.M. The result was a considerable increase in call volume.

The advertising and promotion budget for 1989 was also limited because of expected high demand. Inter+Net paid $50,000 for inclusion of ads in the 11 yellow-pages books produced for 1988–89 in the Washington area. The ads ran under the title "Physicians and Surgeons Information Bureaus."

Exhibit 14.2   Advertisement for Ask-A-Nurse®

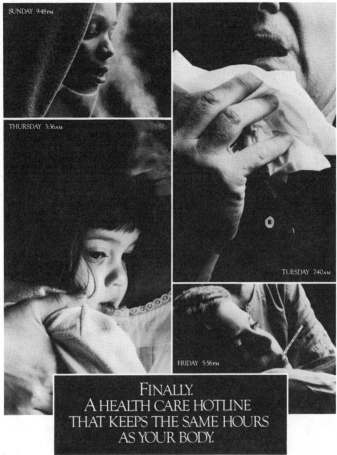

Management believed in 1988 that television advertising of the Ask-A-Nurse system would be needed in 1989 to increase awareness of and interest in the system. Inter+Net Health System planned to spend $272,000 to purchase 30-second ads on three local television stations over 26 weeks. The first 8-week campaign would begin on January 23.

However, the number of calls received in January 1989 averaged 352 a day. An average of 32 calls per day were abandoned by callers after they had been put on hold for more than 20 seconds. Ask-A-Nurse could not hire nurses quickly enough to meet the surge in demand that preceded the television campaign. Concerned that the number of abandoned calls would increase and caller dissatisfaction would rise, Inter+Net Health System managers planned to scale back the television campaign in 1989. No print campaign or other promotion activities were planned.

Callers were routinely asked how they found out about Ask-A-Nurse. In January 1989, 53.5 percent indicated that they were referred by (or heard about the services from) the staff of an Inter+Net hospital. This was a surprise to Inter+Net management, who believed that ads and media attention were the dominant factors in stimulating consumers to call.

Physician Recruitment

To create the data base on physicians, each hospital was given applications for physicians and asked to distribute them. They are expected to keep track of how many physicians enrolled. Physicians signed a form approving the entry of their names into the data base. They had to make decisions on how they would be listed. Some physicians, for example, indicated that they would take Medicare assignments, while others would not. Some were willing to see urgent cases within 24 hours; others would not.

Procedures and Functions

Tasks Carried Out by Nurses

Nurses worked in a large open office, which encouraged interaction among them. Each nurse sat at a desk with a computer terminal and a telephone. Above each desk was a bookshelf with reference books on medicine and maps of communities in the Washington area.

The average call lasted about ten minutes, and the length of the time spent was controlled by the individual nurse. The telephone system in use allowed each nurse to see if one, two, or three calls were on hold. Nurses could then decide whether to shorten their own conversation with a caller.

The system did not require the nurse to read a list of questions, and it did not demand that certain responses be entered before the nurse could move on. Nurses were permitted to leave the record of a call and return later to complete documentation during a time when they were not busy.

The calls that were received could be roughly divided into those where the caller (1) had symptoms or problems or (2) was just seeking information. Either could result in a referral to a physician or medical service. In many cases, no referral was made. The caller could be told to treat the problem at home. The information given might be sufficient to answer the question(s).

Patient Assessment

The nurses used protocols stored in the computer to make an assessment (rather than a diagnosis) of the caller's options if they had a symptom or a perceived medical problem. Sometimes this meant sending the caller to an emergency room; other times it was suggested that the caller wait a day or two and then go to see a physician.

The system assisted the nurses by providing information useful in making an assessment. The protocol for "headache," for example, showed other conditions (for example, vomiting) or circumstances (for example, a recent blow to the head) that would suggest that the problem was emergent.

The protocols were not lists of questions, nor did the nurse enter the answers. Nurses were free to carry on a conversation with the caller, rather than carry out a rigid interview. The nurse entered an assessment into the terminal and used a paper log to show other information that was used in making an assessment, including reference books consulted.

The nurses who worked with Ask-A-Nurse had between 8 and 12 years of experience in nursing. The educational background of nurses at Ask-A-Nurse varied from a masters degree in clinical nursing or health administration to a two-year college degree. The nurses needed a great deal of experience because they had to understand from a set of questions asked by the patient what the problem was and where the patient should go. The protocols in the computer provided useful reminders but did not lead the nurse to a final decision on the advice to give.

Nurses were asked to call back patients who reported symptoms or problems to find out how they were doing, which allowed the patient to discuss their satisfaction with a physician visit or service and allowed the nurse to offer to help again. The computer helped the nurses keep track of who had to be called.

Nurse Satisfaction

Management believed that the nurses liked their work because they could use all of the skills, knowledge, and experience they had in providing help to people, and were free from the administrative responsibilities and politics of a hospital.

The terminals were placed in a single room to allow for the free flow of conversation between nurses. A nurse with a background in psychiatry who got a call concerning a child with a high fever would be able to turn to somebody in the room after placing the patient on hold and ask for assistance in dealing with the problem. This was highly encouraged by management.

Because Ask-A-Nurse was so accessible, the nurses received calls that were medical emergencies. Nurses helped prevent suicides by talking to individuals threatening suicide. They also described how to perform cardiopulmonary resuscitation (CPR) to individuals who had just witnessed a cardiac arrest. The nurses also helped mothers get through a night with a child with a fever and croupy cough, calling them back periodically to see how the child was doing. Although medical emergencies and working all night with a single caller were a small proportion of the work the nurses did, management believed these increased their sense of satisfaction with their jobs.

Referrals

The nurses provided more than information. A nurse might call an ER to tell the staff that a caller had been referred, and what the problem was. A caller who was referred to a physician was asked if they would like the nurse to make an appointment. The telephone system then allowed the nurse to put the caller on hold while an appointment was made, or to initiate a conference call to set up an appointment.

If the caller wanted a referral to a physician, they were asked what they were looking for. The computer stored a large number of characteristics of each physician obtained through a questionnaire. They included the physician's office location, age, sex, length of time in practice, hospital affiliation, board certification, types of insurance accepted, whether the physician expected to be paid in cash at the time of service, and the languages that the physician spoke.

As the caller responded to questions about the importance of these characteristics, the nurse entered the weight (high, medium, or low) that should be given to that characteristic in matching the caller to a physician. The system assumed a medium weight, which the nurse could change to a high or low. The nurses did not ask the caller about the importance of every characteristic. They might skip one or more, depending on whether the caller asked about it and whether the nurse felt it was important given the previous dialogue with the caller. The caller was then told about several (the computer would list up to ten) physicians who met the caller's criteria.

The data stored in the computer could be used to communicate at a later date about other services consumers might be interested in. Mothers of young children, for example, could be sent information on parenting classes. The data base could be searched to select mothers in specific geographic areas with children of a certain age. Inter+Net had not used the data base for this purpose but might carry out such searches for its members in the future. Inter+Net was very concerned, however, about the release of the data, even to its members, because it would violate the confidentiality of its callers.

Hardware and Software

The system operated on a Texas Instruments minicomputer. The Ask-A-Nurse software was an enhancement to Health Match, a program developed by Baxter Healthcare Corporation. The original Health Match software was installed in 250 sites in 1988. Ask-A-Nurse was operating at 52 sites. Inter+Net was a "beta" test site for a new version, Super Health Match (i.e., it was developed at another "alpha" site and has been released to a few others before general release).

The Ask-A-Nurse software contained the protocols for assessing caller symptoms and problems. An organization that bought Ask-A-Nurse obtained a license to use the Health Match program. They could then purchase support and enhancements to both Ask-A-Nurse and Health Match if they so desired.

Evaluation

Management Reports

The Health Match software could automatically produce a series of management reports. For example, the number of calls by age group by day was available through the system, information that could be used to determine the impact of a television ad or newspaper campaign. Baxter also provided a program that allowed managers to format and produce their own reports. Data could also be downloaded in ASCII file format to other report writing and spreadsheet programs.

Management received a separate set of reports from the telephone system that managed incoming calls. The reports showed, for example, the number of calls received, the number of calls processed (i.e., a nurse talked to the caller), and the number of abandoned calls.

Management set a "T-value" for the length of time they believed people would wait before abandoning a call. The T-value used by Inter+Net Health System was 20 seconds. A report showed the number of calls abandoned before and after 20 seconds. The assumption was that people who abandoned a call in less than 20 seconds would frequently call back later. Management believed that when the number of people abandoning a call after 20 seconds increased, it indicated a lack of access that should be investigated and solved by management (for example, by increasing staff at that time period).

The management reports on the telephone system also showed the number of calls handled by each individual nurse, the length of time that nurse was available to take calls, and the average number of staff on duty, as well as the numbers of calls received and the number of calls processed. Reports were available for each hour the system was in operation and for the entire month. This allowed management to determine at what periods of time they were most likely to have calls that they could not handle and when the number of abandoned calls increased, assisting management in setting staffing levels for the various shifts.

Consumer Satisfaction

In addition, Inter+Net obtained information on caller satisfaction when nurses phoned each individual who had a symptom to determine what happened. A formal interview protocol was not used. Callers were asked if they were satisfied with the physician, emergency room (ER), or service they were sent to. If the caller was dissatisfied, a short report was written and sent to the hospital concerned. Hospitals were expected to follow up with their affiliated physicians. If the problem persisted, the physician or service might be dropped from the data base. There were no immediate plans for a formal survey of physicians or callers, and Inter+Net had not asked for vendor support in carrying out a mail or telephone survey.

Characteristics of Callers

About 70 percent of the callers in the first seven weeks had a symptom or problem, or were calling on behalf of someone who did. Callers tended to be younger. There were a large number of mothers calling to discuss their children's problems or seeking information.

Approximately 11 percent of the callers processed in January 1989 indicated they were Medicare beneficiaries, 5 percent were Medicaid, 8 percent were HMO or PPO members, and the remaining 76 percent had other forms of insurance or indicated they would pay for services out-of-pocket.

Feedback to Physicians

A quarterly letter, listing the names of callers referred, was sent to each physician. As indicated earlier, the patient was called to determine what happened. No information was sought from the physician since Inter+Net felt that the response to a physician survey would not be complete or accurate, although comments or criticisms were welcome.

Measuring Impact on Hospital Services

Inter+Net hospitals were to supply the Ask-A-Nurse staff with a computer tape each quarter that provided information on inpatient, outpatient, and ER visits. The Super Health Match software had a program for matching callers with such data. The result would be a report for each hospital that showed the number of visits and admissions, and the revenue received. Hospitals would be able to compare this with their financial contribution to Ask-A-Nurse.

The Ask-A-Nurse staff expected that this matching would not be easy because of the large number of inpatient and outpatient hospital records (more than one million in 12 months) that had to be reconciled to all previous referrals made (more than 50,000 in 12 months). Ask-A-Nurse required that its nurses collect only a small amount of information on each caller—name and address are the minimum. This might make it difficult to match callers to patients.

As of early 1989, Inter+Net had not done a reconciliation of referrals to actual hospital admissions and treatment in the emergency room because of the large volume of data. Other Ask-A-Nurse sites around the country had their hospitals reformat data and submit it on diskettes. The software for this was not part of Super Health Match. Some of the hospitals in the Inter+Net system had complained that they had too many discharges to be able to load the information onto diskettes.

Inter+Net was in the process of buying a tape drive that would be used to read data submitted by Inter+Net hospitals. Super Health Match included a program that uses the information sent by hospitals to create discharge files, which were then matched to referrals.

Growth of the Ask-A-Nurse Program

Inter+Net began operating the Ask-A-Nurse program in September 1988. Even with limited advertising, call volume increased to more than 200 calls per day within seven weeks. A single interview over a local television station resulted in 83 calls within one hour.

By January 1989, call volume averaged 352 per day, making Inter-+Net's Ask-A-Nurse site the busiest in the United States. Of these calls, 320 per day were being processed (i.e., the caller spoke to a nurse). Inter+Net was attempting to hire the additional staff needed to increase the number of calls processed, and to reduce the television advertising that had been planned late in 1988 to run in 1989.

Inter+Net Health System had 14 FTE nurses working at 11 workstations in January 1989. In addition to receiving inbound calls, the nurses were averaging 48 outbound calls per day to arrange physician or hospital appointments and to follow up on patients with symptoms. The average call took 8.6 minutes, but management continued to set five calls per hour as a target to allow for documentation, breaks, and other time not spent on the telephone.

Inter+Net management believed that a service such as Ask-A-Nurse could only be developed in a major metropolitan area by a consortium of hospitals because the high call volume and 24-hour-a-day, seven-day-a-week operation require such a major investment. A single hospital that set up a small system would not be able to handle the call volume and would not have the network of physicians needed to service the people who called.

Why Is Call Volume So High?

Inter+Net Health System had not carried out any studies of why consumers called. Nurses and managers had some impressions which related the response they were seeing to the health care environment in the Washington, D.C., area and nationwide.

First, a significant number of the people who were calling had physicians but were unwilling to call them because they perceived the physician to be very busy. If that were true, why didn't these people talk to the physician's nurse? There had been a significant change in the type of nurse who staffed the physician's office. This individual was rarely a registered nurse, so that patients who might have once called the nurse for advice were more reluctant to do so. The individuals who staffed physician offices were now either medical assistants or LPNs with limited training and experience. A physician would not normally hire a registered nurse because the skills of such a person were not needed.

Second, a number of the people who called asked for a "good general practitioner," which they wanted but couldn't find. Management believed the lack of primary care physicians in the community was responsible for creating part of the demand for Ask-A-Nurse.

Ask-A-Nurse Serves a Midwestern City

Ask-A-Nurse began to serve the Port Huron, Michigan, area under a contract in 1989. The individuals who called the number in Port Huron were not aware that they were calling the Washington, D.C., area. The nurses also did not provide this information.

The hospitals in Port Huron did not have to commit themselves to developing a facility or hiring staff. Inter+Net also benefited by taking advantage of the economies of scale in their current operation. The computer and telephone system could handle more terminals and calls. The marginal cost of buying terminals and other hardware and hiring staff was less than what it would cost to establish a small Ask-A-Nurse site, which would have to be staffed 24 hours a day, seven days a week.

Call volume in Port Huron was not as high as expected, given the size of the area and experience with Ask-A-Nurse elsewhere. One possible explanation was the promotion campaign that had been conducted. The hospitals in the Port Huron area had been doing direct mail advertising, which included 6,000 pieces of direct mail over each week for a three-week period. The response had not been large. Most of the callers had requested a physician, rather than presenting symptoms or requesting a service referral. This suggested that those who called (or referred the caller) were not fully aware of the capabilities of the Ask-A-Nurse system. This might explain the lower response rate.

It was also possible that using direct mail alone did not provide the multiple exposures to the message that produced a response. Consumers in the Port Huron area might just be treating the Ask-A-Nurse promotion as another piece of junk mail. On the other hand, the direct mail strategy might produce a response in the coming weeks and months. Individuals received a magnet with the Ask-A-Nurse number that they could put near their phone. In the future, they might use this number to seek help.

Future Development

Ask-A-Nurse was the first step in the creation of an information center that management hoped would help create a regional health care network. The next step would be to expand the services offered through Ask-A-Nurse and to develop complementary services using a variety of other technologies.

Future of Ask-A-Nurse

Inter+Net management believed that it would have no problem documenting enough admissions and visits to its member hospitals to justify their contributions. The major problem would be to manage the growth of demand for Ask-A-Nurse to assure that callers were answered promptly and received the information they wanted. The amount of advertising that should be done is a major issue since television ads could stimulate much more demand than the current staff could handle.

Inter+Net also faced decisions concerning the use of Ask-A-Nurse by its members. Should the data base be shared, which would allow hospitals to do their own mail and telephone marketing of services? If not, what role should Inter+Net play in promoting the services of an individual member?

Expansion to Other Areas

Inter+Net Health System could enter into contracts with hospitals (as it had already done in Port Huron, Michigan) to provide Ask-A-Nurse services in other areas. It could market its services to the contiguous areas surrounding the Washington, D.C., metropolitan area (for example, Baltimore) or to any area of the United States. Providing Ask-A-Nurse services to a contiguous area, however, might make Inter+Net Health System's services more attractive to employers in the Washington, D.C., area who had employees who lived in those outlying areas or who had satellite locations there.

Inter+Net would benefit from being able to share the fixed costs of operating its Ask-A-Nurse facility with other organizations. Since its marginal costs were low in relation to the costs that would be incurred in developing a new facility, Inter+Net also had the potential to make a profit on such contracts while offering an attractive price.

Offering Other Services through Ask-A-Nurse

Without changing its existing technology, Inter+Net could expand the Ask-A-Nurse system to:

— coordinate home care and case management services

— create and implement specialized triage protocols for dental symptoms, symptoms of persons with malignancies, and women who were pregnant

— provide poison information, integrating its services with the National Capital Poison Control Center to earn grant funding, and funds from corporate sponsors, for both services

— provide benefits information to beneficiaries under a contract with payers, and match them to providers in the Inter+Net Health System who accepted their health insurance

— provide quality assurance services to physicians' practices, hospitals, and outpatient medical centers by contracting with them to conduct standardized surveys over the telephone, or by mail, with their recent patients

— participate in outcomes measurement programs by collecting information from patients recently discharged from Inter+Net Health System hospitals

Several corporations and insurance providers had already contacted Inter+Net Health System to ask whether they could contract with the Ask-A-Nurse facility to provide services to their employees and beneficiaries. Inter+Net management believed that to conceive of Ask-A-Nurse as only a physician referral service was to miss most of the economic opportunities from having registered nurses, a sophisticated data base on medical services in a wide geographical area, and a modern computer and telephone system in one location 24 hours a day.

Telemarketing

When nurses called back people who had symptoms to find out how they were, they got an overwhelmingly favorable response. When people were called who got a referral, but had no symptoms, they did not like it. They asked why the nurse was calling, and whether it was to check up on them. Ask-A-Nurse stopped calling people who were asymptomatic. It had 7,000 calls from people with symptoms in January 1989.

Inter+Net Health System had been the beta test site (i.e., a site for testing prior to general release) for Super Health Match. This product was now changing to become Life Match.™ Life Match would be able to provide data separately for multiple hospitals. This had been a problem, since Inter-+Net Health System wished to report data for its member hospitals separately.

Life Match would also include the "Health Pass" software developed by Baxter Healthcare Corporation. Health Pass allowed a hospital to process health risk appraisal questionnaires and provide reports back to the individual who filled out the form. These individuals could then be approached to participate in various services related to their health concerns or problems.

Life Match would have mass mailing capabilities not currently available in Health Pass. It will also allow power-dialing, that is, the computer would automatically dial the telephone numbers of all people who fit criteria selected by the operator. When someone picked up the telephone, data on that person (including their name, address, and which test they took) would appear on the screen, allowing the operator to individualize a message about services available.

Inter+Net wanted to develop a health promotion and disease prevention program with United Seniors Health Cooperative, an advocacy group for seniors. Seniors would enroll, preferably with their primary care physicians. If they did not have a primary care physician, Ask-A-Nurse would match them with one in the Inter+Net system. Inter+Net would provide a health risk appraisal, which would be scored and a report prepared assessing the need for screening procedures for asymptomatic disease. The report would be prepared by Baxter's Health Pass system. Using Baxter's Life Match system, Inter+Net Health System would periodically mail, depending on their risk factors and need for screening, reminders on which screening procedures they needed to have done.

While this is telemarketing, it is also an attempt to provide good medical care by helping consumers to follow American Cancer Society, and other, recommendations for screening. This made it an extension of the strategy that underlies Ask-A-Nurse, to provide a public service with a payback to the providers who financially support it.

Developing Complementary Services

Inter+Net Health System could also develop complementary services such as the following:

— An answering service for physicians. Operators would have the option of transferring the call to one of the nurses at Ask-A-Nurse. The telephone and computer equipment for an answering service were already installed in the Ask-A-Nurse facility.

— An automated audio text service (see section that follows).

— A computer network that would link member hospitals and affiliated physicians, with an Inter+Net Health System facility serving as the hub of the network. Stored at the hub facility would be data bases. For example, a list of all current beneficiaries could be maintained that could be accessed by hospitals and physicians. The network would also allow for quick transfer of information between physicians and hospitals, for example, notification of a discharge or test results to a physician.

— Inter+Net Health System could use the network just mentioned to collect billing and utilization data and then transmit the bills to third-party payers and/or analyze the data to provide cost, utilization, and outcome reports to members and payers. A direct link to physicians could also speed the correction of errors on claims.

The location of the service and the technology used to handle the request would be transparent (not known and not a problem for) to the caller. A consumer calling a hospital in Maryland would not know that the information they received came from a facility in Virginia. The additional cost of a long-distance call (which would not be borne by the local caller) would be less for a member hospital or a physician to pay than the cost of establishing a similar service.

Automated Audio Text

Using voice recording and transmission technology now available for microcomputers, any audio message could be stored on a computer and then retrieved by anyone with a touch tone telephone. Admitting and discharge procedures at a member hospital could be stored, as well as information on health problems and services (for example, "What is a heart scan?"). The caller could have the option of touching a button to be transferred to the Ask-A-Nurse system.

Inter+Net wanted to create a service bureau for its members. A hospital could rent an hour or two of disk space, make its recordings over the telephone, and change them over the telephone. This could be a complement to Ask-A-Nurse. Callers would be asked whether they wanted to speak to a nurse or get information and could select by pushing the buttons on a telephone. This could be done at the beginning or the end of a call. The service bureau would be at one central location, but callers who dialed a particular hospital would hear a message from that hospital. The location of the service bureau would be transparent to the caller.

Since there were a number of vendors of automated audio text, any competitive advantage could be short-lived. Inter+Net hoped to create a service that its members wanted and offer it at a much lower cost than hospitals would have to pay individually.

Interconnections between Systems

Using both voice and digital communications would allow members, physicians, and consumers a choice in accessing the information in some data bases. A physician who wanted to know preadmission certification procedures for a particular contract could send a message over the computer network or call for an automated audiotape on the procedures. Ask-A-Nurse could be used if questions arose.

Since there were still a number of people who would not (or were afraid to) use a computer, voice communication remained an important choice. The problem was to appropriately train people on which system to use, or interconnect the systems so that Inter+Net Health System staff could help retrieve any information that was requested. A nurse working on Ask-A-Nurse who got a call asking if a patient had been discharged at an Inter+Net hospital could either retrieve the information and provide it to the caller, connect the caller to an automated audiotape system, or transmit the message over a computer link asking a hospital staff member to phone the caller. Inter+Net Health System would leave the caller with the impression that it operated one system committed to service.

Role of Claims Processing

Inter+Net management believed that claims processing and the storage of information on insurance coverage and beneficiaries might be critical to the establishment of Inter+Net as a central information center. If it did not perform these functions, it might be more difficult to persuade physicians to link their computers to a central hub. They might prefer a link to individual hospitals for confidentiality reasons or because they primarily needed insurance and claims information, and to do on-line attestation for Medicare claims.

Management also hoped to link utilization review to the referral of patients, which required data from bills and discharge abstracts. To acquire these data, Inter+Net wanted to begin processing and repricing claims for as many payers as possible.

Management believed that the future for regional health networks was to bypass insurers and contract directly with self-insured employers. Claims processing was an essential step. Inter+Net could then deal directly with the third-party administrator that actually cut the checks, providing claims data that had been edited and repriced. It then built up a very valuable data base to use in negotiations with payers later.

A Partnership with Physicians

Both contracting and the proposed information center would create a complex change in the role of the hospital that could be very threatening to physicians. The hospital's agent—Inter+Net Health System—would take on the roles of performance reviewer (by doing utilization review), claims processor, contract negotiator, and central information source. Physicians would depend on the hospital or its agent for almost all the information essential for the business operations of their practices.

How threatened would physicians actually feel? Inter+Net member hospitals were creating joint ventures between hospitals and physicians, called local provider units or LPUs, to give physicians a greater sense of ownership. The services available through Inter+Net could serve as a powerful inducement for some physicians to join an LPU, and create high switching costs for leaving one.

Implementation

The future developments that have just been outlined had not been approved by Inter+Net's Board of Directors. The developments were desired by individual Inter+Net System managers and board members. The challenge would be to convince the entire board and the constituencies they represented that these particular actions were appropriate and necessary.

Notes

1. Lynn Wagner, "Market Focus—Washington, D.C.," *Modern Healthcare* (November 25, 1988): 34–36, 38.
2. Wagner, "Market Focus," p. 34.
3. Wagner, "Market Focus," p. 34.
4. Wagner, "Market Focus," p. 34.
5. Wagner, "Market Focus," p. 35.

6. Wagner, "Market Focus," p. 35.
7. Wagner, "Market Focus," p. 35.
8. Wagner, "Market Focus," p. 38.
9. Linda Perry, "Hospitals, Doctors Team Up to Gauge HMOs," *Modern Healthcare* (November 18, 1988): 64–66.

Appendixes

Appendix A
Referral One and Service Referral One

APPLICATIONS

1. Physician referral, tracking and follow-up
Referral One can provide the following benefits to your hospital.

A. Promotes referral activities to your physicians, bonding them more closely to your hospital.

Each referral can be documented by an automated, personalized letter to the physician. Additionally, reports on the numbers of referrals to each physician can be printed at regular intervals. These reports show physicians what your hospital is doing for them. They also provide facts which can be useful in management discussions with physicians.

B. Improves efficiency of matching caller needs with physicians.

Compared to a "manual system," Referral One is quicker and far more accurate. Capable of instantaneously matching from one to thirty-one consumer specified criteria with any number of physicians, Referral One removes human error from the matching process. You can customize the system with up to five criteria which are specific to your organization. For example, you could select from all physicians who are participating in a cholesterol reduction program.

C. Improves image of your hospital among callers.

Each caller can be sent a personalized follow-up letter confirming the referral or appointment. These letters can be automatically printed at the end of each day. It is even possible to include a one or two page biography of the physician or a special letter of introduction to the patient from the physician. Combined with your ability to quickly and professionally satisfy consumer needs for a specific physician, these letters will convey your hospital as an efficient, customer-oriented institution.

Source: Reprinted with the permission of National Health Enhancement Systems, Phoenix, Arizona.

253

D. Enforces your standards in rotating referrals among physicians.
Manual systems are inherently subject to operator bias in the referral
process. Automatic rotation of referrals among physicians based on
your pre-established standards is assured by your software. This is the
ideal way to match newcomers with physicians.

**E. Captures information about callers creating a powerful marketing
database.**
Name, address, phone number, age and sex are captured for all callers
as well as insurance coverage and how they heard about your service.
This enables you to analyze the effectiveness of alternative promotional techniques. Additionally, a database is created which can be
used to market other services (e.g., a personalized letter could be sent
to all female respondents announcing a new women's center).

F. Permits better management of physician relations function.
The system tracks referrals to physicians and provides reports which
compare admission revenues to your referral patterns for up to five
years.
    Reports on referrals by speciality can be used to identify staff short-
ages in a speciality helping you identify needs for additional physicians. Other management reports permit you to identify peak call
volume periods, productivity of various staff and geographic patterns
of call activity.

G. Provides a system to permit quality control or other follow-up.
Your staff can follow-up with callers after their initial call to obtain
feedback on whether they saw the physician, their satisfaction and any
other pertinent information impacting future business to your hospital.
For maximum flexibility, the system allows you to select follow-up
calls by referral dates, by next contact date and by demographic
characteristics.
    A "notes" section is established for each caller to your system
providing a historical account of what has been referred to that
caller—and what future follow-up is necessary. Each set of notes can
be coded to facilitate special qualitative reporting such as quality
control of physician care or human interest stories which could lay the
foundation for a marketing campaign.

2. Membership list management and follow-up
Many hospitals are developing membership programs as part of their
marketing strategy. Special memberships your hospital develops can be
pre-loaded on the system. As a person calls in and is interested in becom-

ing a member of your program, you can register them immediately, automatically sending them the appropriate literature.

You can track how they heard about your membership program and produce lists of names and phone numbers, mailing labels and personalized letters on special programs. You can maintain a "notes" file on each member, with a record of all referral and discussion activities. Also, if they need to be re-contacted to market a future program or provide a special service, the follow-up date can be recorded.

Each follow-up activity, whether by telephone or by direct mail, can be targeted based on selected demographics or any other marketing characteristic you track. For example, you may be interested in contacting only those Senior's Program members who responded to a specific media campaign.

3. Physician list management and follow-up

The physician database management capability permits highly targeted communication to your medical staff. The database is also accessible for customized reports you might require. You can identify the number and/or names of all physicians who meet any of 40 different characteristics.

All data collected on physicians is retrievable for personalized mailings to your physicians. For example, you could send a letter about changes in Medicare procedures to all physicians who accept Medicare assignments.

The follow-up capabilities of the physician list management software allow you to systematically manage the physician marketing function. For example:

- A listing of physicians by zip code along with their names, addresses, specialties, phone numbers and admissions information would help your physician relations staff plan productive visits to physicians.

- This same information could lay the foundation for target marketing new or low utilization hospital services to specific groups of physicians.

4. Marketing campaign fulfillment, tracking and follow-up

The system can be used to handle responses to any number of marketing programs. It will provide fulfillment lists for packages to be sent or you can include automated, personalized letters if desired.

Extensive information can be captured on each respondent including name, address, phone, age, sex and how the caller heard of the service as well as additional information which can be customized for your organization. Reports generated can be used to analyze campaign effectiveness.

The data collected also goes into the master marketing data file being created by your system. Thus, it can be accessed for future marketing campaigns.

Tracking of campaigns permits your organization to evaluate the relative effectiveness of alternative marketing approaches. This should prove useful in justifying marketing expenditures.

The system allows for targeted follow-up of individuals, based on demographic or other marketing characteristics you establish. You can produce personalized letters or lists of individuals to call by next contact date, thus making your marketing campaign follow-up timely and effective.

5. Service referral, tracking and follow-up

Service Referral One is designed to be used as a stand-alone system but can be fully integrated with Referral One allowing instant access from one system to the other. The system can coordinate information requests and facilitate referrals including scheduling classes for hospital programs as well as any community services you wish to promote. It is ideal for use by your health education department.

Specific benefits which can be achieved by using Service Referral One include:

A. Positions your hospital as the single source for health information.
Consumers in your market need only to have your phone number to obtain information or obtain referrals to any health related program.

B. Improves image of hospital among callers.
With Service Referral One, you will be able to quickly and efficiently satisfy consumer requests for information. Letters confirming referrals and appointments can be automatically printed at the end of the day.

C. Increases effectiveness of marketing activities.
The system permits the centralization of inquiries about all hospital services. The software allows you to profile your services including complete descriptions, class times, instructors, availability and fee structure. This enables you to answer calls uniformly and in accordance with your pre-established standards.

Also, the caller may have a need for additional services, including a physician referral which can be handled by switching to the physician referral system with a single keystroke.

D. Enables targeted follow-up to maximize effectiveness.
Each person or group of people can be selected for a specific follow-up purpose, whether it be customer satisfaction, getting confirmation of attendance or referring the person to other programs your hospital offers.

Individual notes and next contact date capabilities allow your staff to personalize communications and be punctual in their follow-up efforts, whether by phone or mail.

IMPLEMENTATION

Both systems are designed so they can be operated by small or large providers. For a small organization, existing staff, equipment and facilities can normally be used with the system operating on a single PC. For larger hospitals with multiple stations handling calls, a network version is available.

Getting started

The only equipment needed is a 100% IBM Compatible PC (XT or AT) and access to a printer. Both pieces of equipment can be used for other functions as well.

Installation and training assistance from our personnel is available at your location or in Phoenix. On-going telephone support is provided free for the first twelve months to handle questions or resolve problems related to usage.

Most organizations do not require separate personnel to handle referral calls. The system can be accessed quickly (one keystroke) and the typical call takes just a few minutes. Thus, a secretary, receptionist or administrative assistant could handle referrals along with their other duties.

The physician database can be activated with just four elements of data about each physician: name, specialty, address and phone number. Typically, a user will get started with a minimum of physician information and expand the data at a later date to take full advantage of the system's capabilities.

Generating calls for referrals

Hospitals just getting started in a formal physician referral program may wish to begin with a modest program to generate calls. Existing yellow pages advertising normally can be modified to include a prominent mention of physician referral.

Expanded efforts to generate calls would include single focus referral ads in yellow pages, direct marketing to newcomers and specific physician referral ad campaigns.

In addition, National Health Enhancement Systems has several screening products available which can help feed your physician referral programs. Ask your consultant to provide details.

ECONOMICS

Increased revenue

The financial return realized from using Referral One and Service Referral One will vary based on each organization's economic structure and competitive situation. The following information is intended to provide a basis for potential users to calculate their own financial return.

A. Direct return

Underlying these direct revenue calculations is an assumption that a percentage of patients you refer to physicians will be subsequently admitted to your hospital. This seems reasonable considering most people calling for referrals have a physical problem which could require them to be hospitalized. If your referrals are properly merchandised to a physician, something which Referral One does well with its automatic letters and reports to physicians, the physician should admit the patient to your hospital.

This assumption has been validated by other organizations. A product report published in *Hospitals* magazine by Scripps Memorial Hospital reported a range of admissions from 1 in 12.5 referrals to 1 in 20 referrals. The calculations below assume a similar range.

Assuming an average net contribution of $2,000 per admission and a range of referral calls from 20 per month to 200 per month, the following returns can be projected.

	Admission Revenue Projections		
	20 per Month	*100 per Month*	*300 per Month*
Referrals per year	240	1200	3600
Higher assumption			
Admissions per referral	1/12.5	1/12.5	1/12.5
Admissions	19	96	288
Net contribution per admission* (excluding direct costs of referral program)	$2,000	$2,000	$2,000
Annual contribution	$38,000	$192,000	$576,000
Lower assumption			
Admission per referral	1/20	1/20	1/20
Admissions	12	60	180
Net contribution per admission* (excluding direct costs of referral program)	$2,000	$2,000	$2,000
Annual contribution	$24,000	$120,000	$360,000

*Projected based on deducting direct patient care expenses from net revenues.

Since the system can be used on a part-time basis with no extra FTE's, the payoff for establishing a referral function can be significant in the very first year.

B. Indirect return

Although difficult to measure, the indirect return from using Referral One could be even greater than the direct return.

The system is designed to improve the bonding between a hospital and its physician. It achieves this goal by giving you the opportunity to merchandise your referrals to each doctor by letters and by regular reports.

It stands to reason that the more business you provide each physician, the more loyal he or she become to you. If this does not occur, you will find out from your regular reports comparing admission revenues to referrals and can reallocate your referral priorities.

Sample Reports and Letters

The following is a sample of the reports and letters available from Referral One and Service Referral One.

REFERRAL ONE REPORTS

Physician Profile Review - Detailed information on individual physicians.

Physician Profile Detail - Detailed information on physicians including referral and admissions information.

Physician Profile Summary - Summary of individual physician information including referral and admission information.

Physician Profile - Name and Address - Includes list of physicians by name and address.

Physician Profile - List of physician by ID number, name & phone.

Detail by Physician - List of all callers referred to each individual physician.

Physician Tables - List of physician characteristics being tracked.

Caller List - Address list of all callers.

Caller One Line - Names of callers with date and time of call.

Detail by Caller - Physicians referred, demographic information, letters and packages sent.

Caller Summary - Physicians referred and appointments made for all callers.

Caller Demographic - Caller demographic information.

Caller Tables - List of caller demographics being tracked.

Packages Report - List of materials needed to send to callers.

Log Activity - Activity notes recorded for each caller by time period specified.

REFERRAL ONE LETTERS

Letter to Caller - Listing physicians suggested and appointment scheduled if applicable.

Letter to Physician - Listing callers scheduled for appointments at their offices by date and time.

Physician Monthly Letter - Summarizes all referrals and appointment activity to each physician by month or period specified.

Letter from Physician to Patient - Introduces physician to patient by detailing experience, qualifications, and personal notes if desired.

Custom Letters to Callers - Ability to design your own letters to follow-up with your mailing list of callers regarding special programs and services you offer.

SERVICE REFERRAL ONE REPORTS

Service Profile Review - Detailed information on individual services.

Service Profile Detail - Detailed information on services including referral and enrollment information.

Service Profile Summary - Summary of individual service information including referral and enrollment information.

Service Profile - Name and Address - includes list of services by name and address.

Service Profile - List of services by ID number, name & phone.

Detail by Service - List of all callers referred to each individual service.

Service Tables - List of service characteristics being tracked.

Caller List - Address list of all callers.

Caller One Line - Names of callers with date and time of call.

Detail by Caller - Service referred, demographic information, letters and packages sent.

Caller Summary - Services referred to and enrollments made for all callers.

Caller Demographic - Caller demographic information.

Class Roster - List of class participants for services by date and time.

Caller Tables - List of caller demographics being tracked.

Packages Report - List of materials needed to send to callers.

Log Activity - Activity notes recorded for each caller by time period specified.

SERVICE REFERRAL ONE LETTERS

Letter to Caller - Listing services suggested and enrollment if applicable.

Letter to Service Organization - Listing callers enrolled by class and date.

Letter From Service Director to Caller - Introduces service director and organization to participant by detailing experience, qualifications and personal notes if desired.

Custom Letters to Callers - Ability to design your own letters to follow-up with your mailing list of callers regarding special programs and services you offer.

Appendix B
NHES's Patient Acquisition System

National Health Enhancement Systems, a firm that develops computer software for healthcare marketing, has created a hospital marketing program that combines paper-and-pencil health tests with an integrated outbound telemarketing and direct mail system. The program allows the hospital to identify and target by mail and phone those prospects who have the greatest likelihood of requiring inpatient hospital care in the near future. It also has a tremendous impact from a customer service perception in the hospital's community.

NATIONAL HEALTH'S OUTBOUND TELEMARKETING PROGRAM

Step #1: Hospital Distributes Personal Health Risk Tests to Consumers
The health risk tests—The Heart Test, The Health Test and The Cancer Test—are simple paper-and-pencil "checklists," which consumers fill out themselves. The tests are designed to take a few minutes to complete; questions concern the individual's personal and family medical history, health habits, risk factors and interest in follow-up medical and health promotion programs. In addition, clinical information can be collected by a health professional.

The hospital distributes the tests in direct mailings or newcomer kits or at health fair, blood pressure screenings, physician speaking engagements or physicians' offices. The tests also are short enough to fit into a print advertisement in the local newspaper.

Step #2: Consumers Return Tests to the Hospital for Scoring
The hospital offers to evaluate each consumer's test responses at no charge, or for a nominal charge if a clinical component is included.

Step #3: Hospital Scores Tests and Mails Personalized Results to Each Participant
Hospital telemarketers enter the test responses into a computer database; a software package scores each test on the basis of these responses. Participating consumers receive a computer-generated report containing a number score that describes their risk of devel-

Source: Reprinted with the permission of National Health Enhancement Systems, Phoenix, Arizona.

oping a certain health disorder, such as heart disease. The report concludes with a customized "call to action" referral section. For example, this section might prompt the consumer to change his or her diet, see a physician or call a hospital number for service referral.

Step #4: Hospital Selects Individuals at High Risk of Developing Health Disorder for Outbound Telemarketing
The hospital telemarketing staff selects groups of individual participants for follow-up based on age, sex, health risk scores, need for personal physician and/or other criteria appropriate to the hospital's product line. Two examples follow.

Example #1
The hospital selects all males who participated in a corporate health screening who are between the ages of 30 and 60, who are key managers, who are at higher than average risk of heart disease and who are interested in finding a doctor and having a medical check-up.

Example #2
The hospital selects all females who responded to a particular mailing who are between the ages of 25 and 60, who are interested in women's programs and in being referred to a family physician, who had reported on the health risk test symptoms not discussed with a physician and who have not seen a physician for at least three years.

Step #5: Hospital Telemarketers Place Calls to Selected Individuals
The software program produces telemarketing scripts based on the service(s) that the hospital wants to sell to a particular consumer. For example, the script for cardiovascular services leads the telemarketer through a call to an individual at high risk for heart disease. The telemarketer describes the potentially alarming test results as an "opportunity" for the individual to take preventive measures immediately.

Step #6: Telemarketers Sell High-Risk Individuals Clinical Assessment and Fitness Programs and Physician Referrals
The telemarketing script is designed to persuade the individual to see a physician or come into the hospital for a follow-up health assessment. The assessment, also designed by National Health, can utilize existing hospital resources and include a treadmill test, a blood analysis and counseling. Hospital profits on the assessment range between 40% and 60%.

In addition to the follow-up clinical assessment, telemarketers often refer consumers to stress management programs, stop smoking classes, regular blood pressure and cholesterol checks, weight reduction programs, nutritional counseling or supervised exercise programs. Telemarketers also offer participants a physician referral. In past health risk test screenings, 20% to 40% of the screened individuals did not have a primary care physician.

The substantial revenues to be derived from the health risk test screenings, however, would result from the generation of inpatient admissions. While none of the participating hospitals has yet documented a large number of admissions directly attributed to the program, potential inpatient revenues are presented below.

FINANCIAL IMPACT

The Patient Acquisition System can generate substantial revenue—both direct and indirect—for your institution.

Of course, the amount of revenue can vary considerably, depending upon your institution and how you use the PAS. Some of the factors influencing revenue include:

- the services and programs offered at your institution;
- your institution's rate structure;
- the avenues through which you distribute questionnaires;
- your target audience for the PAS;
- the volume of screenings you achieve; and
- the type and effectiveness of your follow-up activities.

But to get an idea of what you might expect from the PAS, let's take a look at a typical full-service, acute-care hospital. Let's say this hospital plans to use the PAS mainly as a way of increasing referrals to their physicians.

Based on these assumptions, this hospital can expect gross, direct referral revenue of $662,250 and net contribution to fixed costs and profit of $297,000 during the first year. The direct incremental costs to operate this system are approximately $68,000 during year one, with $38,400 attributable to direct labor costs.

If this hospital can tap into existing labor resources, the contribution to fixed costs and profit will increase proportionately. The hospital's physicians will also benefit from the follow-up activity at an estimated amount of $293,000, assuming the organization has an open heart surgical program. (See Exhibit D_3: Gross Revenue—Direct Referrals.)

These are the direct financial benefits that you can expect as a result of PAS. But there are also indirect financial revenues, which may prove to be equally, if not more, important to the long-term success of your organization.

1. The PAS enables you to build corporate services.

The PAS offers you an excellent opportunity to establish and build relationships with corporate America. You can begin by offering to screen a company's employees with The Heart Test or The Health Test. This can be done free of charge, as a loss leader, or you can combine the questionnaire with a low-cost clinical screening, such as a cholesterol check.

By doing such a screening, you establish the opportunity to discuss with company executives, the management summary reports and then to propose follow-up wellness programs or diagnostic services for the company. With today's spiraling health care costs, many corporations are looking for proactive ways to reduce their employee health care benefit costs. Some franchises have even established worksite clinics at local companies. Other possibilities include managed care contracts, occupational medicine services and employee assistance programs.

Thus, the PAS can lead to a long-term, service-oriented relationship between your organization, your physicians and local companies. And NHES will help you get started with The Corporate Account Lead Generation Program.

2. The PAS builds community image and programs.

In today's crowded marketplace, it is becoming harder and harder to get positive public exposure. The PAS offers an effective way to create public interest and to educate the public about your institution's services and programs.

The questionnaires can be distributed via your organization's speakers bureau, community health fairs, publications, physicians' offices. And, when the questionnaires are dovetailed with an activity about a particular product line (your cancer, heart or diabetes center, for example), the PAS can be a particularly effective way to inform the public about your services.

In addition to informing the public about your institution, the questionnaires provide you with a valuable source of potential patients. Timely follow-up with respondents results in increased use of your programs and services.

3. The PAS extends marketing dollars.

Your marketing department probably coordinates many events and activities that could be enhanced by the PAS questionnaires. By distributing the questionnaires at these events, you can track participation in your marketing efforts and turn these events into referral generators.

As a PAS franchise, you will avoid the high costs associated with the development and maintenance of a health screening product system. And you'll be able to obtain high quality promotional materials at the lower costs available through the large scale buying power of a national network.

4. The PAS enables you to build a marketing database.

The PAS questionnaires allow you to collect a wealth of valuable information on potential customers: demographics, insurance coverage, potential health problems and medical interests. With this information, you can establish and continually build a marketing database.

This database enables you to promote your hospital's services and programs to individuals who have a need for and/or interest in specific programs. And, you can use the information in your database to develop new programs and services, and to effectively publicize existing ones.

5. The PAS links you to a national network of health care providers.

As a PAS franchise, you will have access to specialists in corporate marketing, community relations, computer technology, telemanagement, and research and development. The NHES team works to provide state-of-the-art marketing technology and service to all our franchises. Our professionals are always just a phone call away.

Being part of the NHES network will also enable you to share ideas, problems and solutions with other PAS providers from across the country.

Acquiring the PAS is an excellent step toward planning for the short- and long-range financial success of your institution.

NOTE: Any revenue or profit projections made in the section above are not to be construed as an earnings claim. National Health Enhancement makes no claim as to the potential earnings resulting from the purchase of a franchise.

Exhibit D₁ Data Base Profile Results from an Exemplary Heart and Cancer Screening Program

Heart Test Screening Results		
Description	Estimated Number	Percentage
Total people screened	10,000	100%
Average age—50 years old		
Family history/heart disease	4,700	47%
Personal history/heart disease	1,300	13%
High blood pressure	1,400	14%
Severely overweight: 25 pounds	3,200	32%
High risk	1,500	15%
High moderate risk	1,800	18%
Interest in physician	1,500	15%
Interest in medical exam	3,000	30%
Interest in risk reduction	4,000	40%
Interest in weight management	5,000	50%
Interest in stop smoking	1,200	12%
Interest in stress reduction	3,500	35%

Cancer Test Screening Results		
Description	Estimated Number	Percentage
Total people screened	10,000	100%
Average age—53 years old		
Has warning signs of cancer	1,800	18%
Interest in physician	1,200	12%
Interest in medical exam	3,200	32%
Interest in risk reduction	3,300	33%
Interest in weight reduction	3,700	37%
Cancer check-up recommended:		
*Medical examination	6,800	68%
*Digital rectal	5,200	52%
*Stool blood test	4,600	46%
*Proctosigmoidoscopy	4,200	42%
*Prostate examination	2,400	24%
*Testicle examination	2,400	24%
*Mammogram	2,800	28%
*PAP test	1,400	14%

Exhibit D₂ Financial Impact—Net Contribution to Fixed Costs and Profits: Direct Referrals Only (excluding program acquisition costs)

Description	Exhibit	Year 1	Year 2	Year 3	Year 4	Year 5	Total
Gross direct referral revenue	*	$662,250	$688,740	$716,290	$744,941	$774,739	$3,586,960
Incremental direct operating costs:	*						
Labor (assumes additional staff)		38,400	41,472	44,790	48,373	52,243	225,277
Promotional materials & participant reports		22,100	23,868	25,777	27,840	30,067	129,652
Other		7,700	8,316	8,981	9,700	10,476	45,173
Total		68,200	73,656	79,548	85,912	92,785	400,102
Net contribution to fixed costs and profit— excluding direct patient care expense		594,050	615,084	636,741	659,029	681,953	3,186,857
Less: Marginal costs for direct patient care (50%)		297,025	307,542	318,371	329,514	340,977	1,593,429
Net contribution to fixed costs and profits		$297,025	$307,542	$318,371	$329,514	$340,977	$1,593,429
Note: Adjustment for reduced labor cost assuming existing staff		(38,400)	(41,472)	(44,790)	(48,373)	(52,243)	(225,277)
Net adjusted contribution to fixed costs and profit		$335,425	$349,014	$363,160	$377,887	$393,220	$1,818,706

*Refer to following schedules in this exhibit series.

Exhibit D₃ Gross Revenue—Direct Referrals

Description		Number	Average Hospital Revenue	Total Estimated Hospital Revenue	Average Physician Revenue	Total Estimated Physician Revenue
People screened (all screening products)	Note 1*	10,000				
People contacted for risk & interest follow-up	Note 2*	3,500				
People referred to physicians	Note 3*	1,650				
People who kept appointments		990			$175	$173,250
People referred to other hospital programs	Note 4*	350	$225	$78,750		
People referred to outpatient procedures by physicians	Note 5*	150	$450	$67,500		
Inpatient admissions:	Note 6*	66				
General medical/surgical (85%)		56	$4,750	$266,000	$800	$44,800
Cardiovascular surgery (15%)		10	$25,000	$250,000	$7,500	$75,000
Total gross revenue				$662,250		$293,050

*Refer to attached revenue assumptions.

Exhibit D$_4$
Revenue Assumptions

1. Projections are based on a recommended implementation model in which each franchise screens 10,000 participants annually;

2. Assumes respondents who are at high risk and high/moderate risk are contacted along with those who are interested in a medical evaluation or securing a physician;

3. Assumes that 50% of the respondents contacted will be referred to a new or current physician and that 60% of those referred (990) will keep the appointment. Assigns an average revenue value of $175 for each physician encounter assuming the range of fees to be $75–$300 depending on visit type and whether care is provided by primary or specialty care physicians;

4. Assumes that 10% of the respondents contacted will be referred to a specific intervention program such as weight management, smoking cessation, stress management at an average fee of $225 according to NHES estimates.

5. The Health Care Advisory Board in their June 1988 publication indicated that approximately 9% of physician referrals resulted in subsequent outpatient procedures at an average gross revenue of $400;

6. The Health Care Advisory Board in their June 1988 study indicated that their average in-patient revenue was $4,000 and that up to 7% of physician referrals resulted in hospitalization. For purposes of this pro forma, a 4% in-patient admission rate was used. These estimates do not reflect in-patient admission revenue associated with cardiovascular surgery and cardiac catheterization which would logically follow as a by-product of screening 10,000 people with The Heart Test questionnaire. The physician revenue associated with in-patient admissions reflects the aggregate professional fees for all doctors involved in the care of hospitalized patients.

Exhibit D₅ Incremental Direct Operating Costs

Description		Unit Quantity	Unit Cost	Additional Staff	Existing Staff
Incremental direct labor costs:					
Health coordinator (elective—1 FTE)	Note 1*			$30,000	$0
Data entry clerical support (part time, 1, 200 hrs @ $7.00)	Note 2*			8,400	0
Total incremental direct labor				38,400	0
Promotional materials and participant reports:					
Screening questionnaires (average assortment of types)	Note 3*	30,000	0.20	6,000	6,000
Report forms (average assortment of types)	Note 4*	10,000	1.25	12,500	12,500
Direct mail campaigns (mailing list, postage & processing)	Note 5*	10,000	0.36	3,600	3,600
Total				22,100	22,100
Other:					
Training in Phoenix (approximate—will vary by site)	Note 6*			1,200	1,200
Support fees (approximate—may vary by site)	Note 7*			5,000	5,000
Miscellaneous (approximate—office supplies, etc.)				1,500	1,500
Total				7,700	7,700
Total direct incremental costs (excluding acquisition costs)				$68,200	$29,800

*Refer to attached cost assumption.

Exhibit D$_6$
Cost Assumptions

1. Assumes 1 FTE health coordinator to oversee the delivery of the entire program. In those cases where a hospital is organized to disseminate the distribution and follow-up activities, the full-time effort of the health coordinator can be spread among operating departments;

2. Assumes clerical support is needed to enter completed screening questionnaires and process participant reports. An alternative to paid clerical support is the use of hospital volunteers or NHES' Service Bureau;

3. Assumes that of the 30,000 questionnaires, 10,000 are disseminated via direct mail campaigns. The balance are distributed through health screening engagements, speaking bureaus, occupational medicine contracts, etc.;

4. Assumes the average report fee plus postage is approximately $1.25. The report only fee ranges between $.90–$1.50.

5. Assumes the per unit cost includes mailing list acquisition, bulk postage and mailing house processing;

6. Assumes an average per person expense of $1,200 to cover travel and lodging while in training, in Phoenix, Arizona;

7. Support fees paid to NHES will vary with the population of the exclusive market territory.

8. Exhibit D$_2$ assumes expense in years 2–5 will increase an average of 8% per year.

Exhibit D₇   The Heart Test™ Screening Results—Various Sites

Location Dates	Hypothetical Projection	Actual Results					
		San Jose 6/87–8/87	Lafayette, LA 10/87	Laguna Hills, CA 1/88–5/88	St. Louis, MO 9/87–5/88	Indianapolis, IN 2/87–3/88	Chattanooga, TN 9/88
Total screened		1022	1503	724	2523	1061	1548
Average age	50	49	48	50	45	52	46
% Incidence of:							
High risk	15%	23%	16%	18%	12%	23%	22%
High moderate risk	18%	17%	18%	20%	14%	22%	18%
Total higher risk	33%	40%	34%	38%	26%	45%	40%
% Interested in:							
Compreh. medical exam	32%	33%	78%	35%	47%	62%	32%
Compreh. cardio. exam	30%	34%	NA	NA	NA	NA	43%
Reducing risk of heart attack/stroke	40%	27%	73%	55%	51%	63%	86%
Family M.D. or specialist	15%	18%	NA	12%	2%	NA	26%
Weight management	50%	50%	73%	37%	52%	61%	47%
Stop smoking	12%	16%	18%	7%	13%	19%	17%
Stress reduction program	35%	41%	20%	12%	47%	60%	39%

THE HEART TEST™

A RISK FACTOR ANALYSIS

Please print clearly

Social Security # _____

Name _____
Last   First   MI

Address _____

Zip Code _____ City _____ State _____

Telephone: Day (___) _____ Eve. (___) _____

Age ____ Birthdate ___/___/___ Sex ____ Today's Date ___/___/___

Type of health coverage: (check all that apply)

HMO ____ PPO ____ Major Medical ____ Medicare/Medicaid ____ None ____

Other ____ Name of Insurance Co. _____

Race ____ (1) Caucasian   (2) Black   (3) Hispanic   (4) Oriental
(5) American Indian   (6) Other

Height ____ ft. ____ in.   Weight: _____ lbs.   (S·A)

Please answer ALL questions. Write your "point score" in each box.

1. Age/Sex:	Male—Age	51 and over	10	
		35 - 50	6	
		34 and under	1	☐
	Female—Age	51 and over	5	
		35 - 50	2	
		34 and under	0	

2. Family History:	If you have parents, brothers, or sisters who have had a heart attack, stroke, or heart bypass surgery		
	At age 59 or BEFORE	5	
	At age 60 or AFTER	3	☐
	None of the above or don't know	0	

3. Personal History:	If you have had a heart attack	20	
	If you have not had a heart attack but have had angina, heart bypass surgery, angioplasty, stroke or blood vessel surgery	10	☐
	None of the above	0	

4. Smoking:	CURRENT cigarette smoker:		
	and you smoke 25 or MORE cigarettes a day	10	
	and you smoke 24 or LESS cigarettes a day	5	
	PREVIOUS cigarette smoker within last TWO years:		☐
	and you smoked 25 or MORE cigarettes a day	5	
	and you smoked 24 or LESS cigarettes a day	3	
	Never smoked or quit smoking more than TWO YEARS ago	0	

5. High Blood Pressure:	If you have had your blood pressure taken in the LAST YEAR		
	and it was Elevated or High	6	
	and it was Borderline	3	☐
	and it was Normal	0	
	None of the above or don't know	N	

6. Diet:	Which of the following best describes your eating pattern:		
	One serving of red meat and/or fried foods daily, more than seven eggs a week, and daily consumption of butter, whole milk and cheese	6	
	Red meat four to six times weekly, four to seven eggs weekly, some margarine, low fat dairy products, cheese and/or fried foods	3	☐
	Poultry, fish, little or no red meat, three or less eggs weekly, some margarine, skim milk, and skim milk products	0	

© National Health Enhancement Systems, Inc.   *[Continued]*

	Points	Score

7. Diabetes: Have you ever been told that you have diabetes?
YES at age 40 or **BEFORE** .... (Male 3 - Female 6)
YES at age 41 or **AFTER** .... (Male 2 - Female 4)
NO 0

8. Weight: Please enter your height and weight.

Height [ft. | in.]   Weight [lbs.]

Your score will be calculated for you

9. Exercise: Do you engage in any aerobic exercise such as brisk walking, jogging, bicycling, racquetball, or swimming for more than 15 minutes:
Less than ONCE a week 3
ONE to TWO times a week 1
THREE or more times a week 0

10. Stress: How well do the following traits describe you:
COMPETITIVE, BOSSY, EASILY ANGERED, PRESSED FOR TIME.
VERY WELL 6
FAIRLY WELL 3
NOT AT ALL 0

11a. How many YEARS since your last complete medical evaluation?

11b. Check this box if you have a physician with whom you can discuss the results of this test.

Health Interests: (S-A)
Check which of the following health areas would be of interest to you or your spouse.

	Yes	
Interested In:	**Self**	**Spouse**
12. Family Doctor or Specialist	☐	☐	12.
13. Comprehensive Medical Checkup	☐	☐	13.
14. Comprehensive Cardiovascular Evaluation	☐	☐	14.
15. Blood Pressure/Cholesterol Check	☐	☐	15.
16. Reducing Risk of Heart Attack/Stroke	☐	☐	16.
17. Weight Management Program	☐	☐	17.
18. Stress Management Program	☐	☐	18.
19. Cancer Risk Reduction Program	☐	☐	19.
20. Stop Smoking/Tobacco Stoppers Program	☐	☐	20.
21. Fitness Assessment/Custom Exercise Program	☐	☐	21.
22. Seniors' Programs	☐	☐	22.
23. Women's Health Programs	☐	☐	23.
24. Low Back Care	☐	☐	24.

To be completed by a physician or health professional (OPTIONAL)

25. Height _____ in.
26. Weight _____ lbs.
27. Blood Pressure _____ / _____ mmHg
28. Body Fat _____ %
    Sum 3 Site _____ mm
    Sum 7 Site _____ mm

29. Total Cholesterol _____ mg/dl
30. HDL Cholesterol _____ mg/dl
31. LDL Cholesterol _____ mg/dl
32. Triglycerides _____ mg/dl
33. Blood Glucose _____ mg/dl
34. Max VO2 _____ ml/kg/min

Appendix C

CENTRAL CONTACT SYSTEM^{SM}

MODULE DESCRIPTIONS

PHYSICIAN REFERRAL Module:

The Physician Referral Module helps market your physicians to the community. This system matches the client to the right physicians based on their needs, preferences, and physician loyalty.

The Central Contact System prints follow-up letters to the client as well as monthly reports to the physician. This easy to use system is the mainstay in every good healthcare marketing effort.

HEALTHCARE SERVICES REFERRAL Module:

This system helps register clients for classes, such as Weight Management or Stop Smoking. In addition the system can refer clients to substance abuse, mental health or any other like programs.

This module will also print follow-up letters and monthly management reports.

MARKETING CAMPAIGN, LITERATURE FULFILLMENT Module:

This system is used to track the effectiveness of marketing campaigns and to send additional information to the client concerning any of your programs.

When a person sends in a request or calls in response to an advertisement, the system tracks where, when, what & how the client contacted you. Then additional information can be sent to the client.

Summary Reports are available to help show what marketing efforts are paying off.

BUSINESS AND INDUSTRY Module:

This module allows you to track your marketing efforts to businesses and industry. It provides stronger control over the sales process and timely reports for management review.

The system can automate the tasks of organizing your clients, help analyze the information and provide a valuable decision making tool.

PHYSICIAN RELATIONS Module:

This system is used to help manage the relations between the hospital and your medical community, both physicians ON STAFF and those NOT ON STAFF.

Speciality, practice type, needs, interest and other relevant information is stored to allow proper follow-up and interface with your medical community.

MODULE DESCRIPTIONS

MEMBERSHIP TRACKING Module:

This module can help track the various membership programs that you have at the hospital. Direct Mail letters and mailing labels can be produced, saving hours of work now done by hand. Any group can be targeted for a phone call and by using the TELEMARKETING SCRIPTS option you can contact them about a new program or service that might interest them.

MATERNITY CLUB Module:

The Maternity Club module is designed to register mothers who are expecting along with their physicians name, etc. The software then allows you to print a letter or label to each expectant mother, based on their due date.

Monthly you can send information about their pregnancy, care of the child, or related hospital services that they may need.

SENIOR MEMBERSHIP & HOSPITAL UTILIZATION Module:

If your hospital has a Senior Membership Program or you are interested in starting one, this module will help with the administrative task of managing the program.

You can track membership demographics, physician, insurance and other relevant items about each of your members. You can also track the utilization of hospital services by each Senior Member.

FUND RAISING / CHARITABLE CONTRIBUTION Module:

Keep track of those charitable contributions and pledges and let the system handle the administrative tasks for you.

The system will print end of year statements for the contributor as well as reminder notices for those pledges not yet collected.

As with the other systems, when you need to send a letter to each contributor next year you can do it with a few keystrokes.

CENTRAL CONTACT SYSTEM^{SM}   FUNCTIONS & FEATURES

* CENTRAL CONTACT SYSTEM allows you to keep track of all your clients with ease. These include clients YOU need to keep to improve your marketability: membership lists; direct sales contacts; direct mailing lists; inbound/outbound telemarketing; and many other client groups.

 * The FORM LETTER selection allows you to write "FORM LETTERS" once. You can then personalize each letter with any or all clients' names and addresses on it. This can save you many hours of typing and at the same time lets each client feel important.

 * The TELEMARKETING module is included which allows you to write scripts about your various programs and/or products. These scripts can then be used to provide consistent, current information to your clients during phone follow-up or cold calls.

 * TASK SCHEDULING is built into the CENTRAL CONTACT SYSTEM allowing you to define a set of steps to be taken with any given client. TASK SCHEDULING will then prompt you at each appropriate time and date with the exact steps to be taken. The task module helps to ensure timely and accurate follow-up is being given to each of your clients. TASK SCHEDULING also allows you to record estimated time, revenue and expenses that each task should take. Once each task is completed, any notes can be recorded concerning the task along with the actual time spent, revenues, expenses, date task is completed and the person who performed the task.

 * MANAGEMENT REPORTS are provided to allow you to see what tasks are completed and what tasks are left to be done, if any. MANAGEMENT REPORTS also allows you to track each person who uses the system for productivity in a report that is easy to understand.

* The TO/DO option prompts you each morning with the tasks that need to be completed that day along with any tasks that are past due.

* The REPORTS MODULE gives you over 40 standard reports that are included and can be printed. The reports can be either detailed or in summary form. In addition, you can easily create and print your own personalized reports and mailing labels (1,2,3 across).

* A simple to learn TEXT EDITOR is provided, allowing you to write letters, Telemarketing Scripts and add new data fields to your screens.

* HELP SCREENS are included to aid you with online information in using the system. At most points in the software if you need further information about a data item or a particular function, simply press the HELP KEY and additional information will be displayed for your review.

* MULTIPLE SALES PEOPLE AND PCs can be used, as the software is designed to handle the multiple salesperson office, or multiple PCs situation. It has extensive Import/Export capabilities to help transfer information into and out of your office system.

* SYSTEM REQUIREMENTS:
Minimum
Hardware: IBM PC, XT, AT or 100% compatible, 640k memory, 20mb hard disk, and Monochrome or Color Monitor. (286 processor recommended)
Software: DOS 3.1 or higher
Printer : 80, 132 column dot matrix or HP LaserJet.
Network : Software is network compatible with Novell™ Netware.

Appendix D

SYSTEM OVERVIEW

THE OPERATING ROOM SCHEDULING OFFICE SYSTEM

ORSOS, the Operating Room Scheduling Office System, is the state of the art surgical department management information system which utilizes microcomputers in helping surgical departments increase their effectiveness and efficiency through better information handling.

ORSOS is made up of four integrated modules.

- **SCHEDULER** automates the appointment book, including sophisticated conflict checking. It also produces schedules, case records, the OR Log, and daily statistics on demand.

- **REPORTER** summarizes the statistics for each month and year-to-date with management reports and graphs.

- **INVENTORY** provides preference cards, full inventory control, charge capturing, implant log, supply requistions and cost reporting.

- **CONTROLLER** maintains all system data relating to staff members, rooms, procedures, surgeon privileges and major equipment.

All modules are integrated by sharing a central database employing state-of-the-art software. Customized screen formats and reports can be generated quickly on demand.

ORSOS MAIN MENU

```
        (1)     SCHEDULER
        (2)     SCHEDULER REPORTS
        (3)     CONTROLLER
        (4)     INVENTORY
        (5)     INVENTORY REPORTS
        (6)     CHARGE INTERFACE
        (7)     REPORTER
        (8)     REPORT WRITER
        (9)     PERIOPERATIVE
        (10)    PERSONNEL SCHEDULING
        (11)    WORD PROCESSING

        (7)     BACKUP DATA
        (8)     ARCHIVE
        (9)     UTILITIES
        (10)    EXIT ORSOS and return to DOS




Enter item number:
```

Source: Excerpted from John Holton, *ORSOS* (San Jose, California: Atwork Corporation, 1989), with permission.

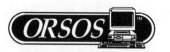

THE BASE SYSTEM
MODULE OVERVIEW

CONTROLLER

STAFF
PROCEDURES
RESOURCES
BLOCKS AVAILABLE
PRIVILEGES
ANESTHESIA AVAILABLE
ROOMS
ENCUMBRANCES

SCHEDULER

APPOINTMENT BOOKING

ADMISSION REPORT
CASE RECORD SHEET
DAILY OR SCHEDULES
DAILY OR LOG
DAILY STATSTICS

DAILY ASSIGNMENT
WORKSHEET

Patient's
ORSOS
Record

INVENTORY

PREFERENCE CARDS
INVENTORY CONTROL
VENDOR PROFILE
INSTRUMENT TRAYS
IMPLANT LOG
CHARGE CAPTURE
SUPPLY REQUISITIONS
SUPPLY RECEIVING
INVENTORY RECORDS

REPORTER AND REPORT WRITER

YEAR-TO-DATE REPORTS

PERIODIC REPORTS

SPECIAL STUDIES

REPORT GENERATOR

SYSTEM SECURITY

All of the modules in *ORSOS* are password-protected for the security of the system. To enter into each module, the user must type in the Password and User ID number. This provides every update with an ID number, user's initials, and a date and time stamp that provides an audit trail.

PASSWORD SCREEN

```
(1) THE PASSWORD:     XXXXXXXX

(2) ORSOS OPERATOR 558-84-8707    MILLER, ELIZABETH

(3) DATE: 10/03/85

(4) TIME: 14:03




    Enter item number:
```

OTHER HIGHLIGHTS

In addition:

- All modules are password protected.
- There is no advance booking time limit imposed by the system. Cases can be booked as far in advance as desired.
- All data is backed up and archived, and is easily restored.
- "HELP" keys provide on-line user assistance when needed.
- *ORSOS* can be networked so that more than one user can work simultaneously, with records available to only one user at a time.
- *ORSOS* can be integrated with other hospital computer systems including financial and materials management.

Each module, with its associated reports and worksheets, is briefly described in the sections that follow.

CONTROLLER

The CONTROLLER

- Maintains the data base for *ORSOS*
- Provides on demand listings of all data in a variety of formats.

CONTROLLER FUNCTION MENU

```
    (1)     UPDATE STAFF RECORDS
    (2)     UPDATE PHYSICIAN PRIVILEGES
    (3)     UPDATE PROCEDURES
    (4)     UPDATE ROOMS
    (5)     UPDATE RESOURCES
    (6)     UPDATE BLOCK TIMES
    (7)     UPDATE ENCUMBRANCES
    (8)     UPDATE AVAILABLE ANESTHESIA

    (9)     LIST STAFF RECORDS
   (10)     LIST PHYSICIAN PRIVILEGES
   (11)     LIST PROCEDURES
   (12)     LIST ROOMS
   (13)     LIST RESOURCES
   (14)     LIST BLOCK TIMES
   (15)     LIST ENCUMBRANCES
   (16)     LIST AVAILABLE ANESTHESIA

 Enter item number:
```

The CONTROLLER maintains the permanent data elements of the system and on-demand listings of the databases sorted in a variety of ways. Data is collected on the following:

- **Operating Rooms** - including off-site facilities such as Labor and Delivery and ambulatory surgical centers.

- **Staff Members** - each staff member, surgeon, anesthesiologist, or other professional scheduled for a case.

- **Surgical Procedures** - with service codes, set-up and clean-up times, and ICD-9 codes.

- **Resources** - includes all major equipment whose unavailability would cause a case cancellation or delay.

- **Blocks** - describes available blocktime for a service, surgeon, or group.

- **Privileges** - indicates the privilege status granted, e.g. full, proctor required, suspension, etc., for each surgeon for each procedure.

- **Encumbrances** - stores scheduling reminders that equipment, rooms, or personnel cannot be scheduled at selected times. Used for equipment maintenance, vacations, conferences, staff meetings etc.

- **Anesthesia** - includes the schedules for each anesthesia staff member. This information is incorporated into the Appointment Book.

SCHEDULER

The SCHEDULER:

- Automates the scheduling of cases with complete conflict checking.
- Produces admission records, surgery schedules, case records and case logs on demand.
- Allows the collection of comprehensive data on each case.
- Provides fast "lookup" of a surgeon's cases, room utilization, equipment reserved, etc.
- Facilitates the case assignments of surgical personnel.
- Prepares daily statistics automatically.
- Waiting List stores patient information about potential surgical cases without requiring a schedule date.
- Real Time Scheduling provides dynamic scheduling changes and feeds the *ORSOS* schedule monitors which automate the "big board".
- ADT Download transfers patient demographic information from your hsopital mainframe to *ORSOS*.

SCHEDULER FUNCTION MENU

```
        (1)   APPOINTMENT BOOK
        (2)   ALTER CASE DATA
        (3)   REAL TIME SCHEDULING
        (4)   ADT ATLINK

        (5)   PRINT DAILY SCHEDULE (short form)
        (6)   PRINT DAILY SCHEDULE (long form)
        (7)   PRINT CASE REPORT
        (8)   PRINT DAILY LOG
        (9)   DAILY STATISTICS
       (10)   ADMISSION REPORT
       (11)   DAILY ASSIGNMENT WORKSHEET
       (12)   REPORT DATA CHECKER



    Enter item number:
```

APPOINTMENT BOOK SCREEN

```
(1)WORK/DT:          (2)RM:      (3)TM:    CASE:      0
(4)SURGEON:                                (7)PAT:
(5)ASST SURGEON:                           (8)PROCEDURE:
(6)RESIDENT:                               (9)PROCEDURE:
(10)Appointment Book DATE:  12/02/86   |DOW:  TUE
-----------------------------------------------------------------------------
     CYSTO    OR#1       OR#2       OR#3       OR#4      OR#5       OR#6
-----------------------------------------------------------------------------
a    07:30    07:30      07:30      07:30      07:30     07:30      07:30
      |      |SPOHRER, G GRIFFIN, P|UROL      |HOLTON,  J NESS, A   WARNER,  M
      |      |PACE INSER C-SECTION |          |PACE INSER ESOPHAGOSC RHINOPLAST
      |_____|MASSEY,BIL SPOONER,CI|_____|CLIFFORD,A LARSON,SCO BLOCK,ROBT

b             09:33      08:55      12:15      09:33     10:05      09:20
      |      |           GRIFFIN, P HOLTON, J  WARNER,  D SPOHRER, G JOHNSON, J
      |      |           D&C        C-SECTION  AMPUT FING CHIN IMPLT AMPUT FING
      |_____|           MOON,CATHY HORNING,G  LEMIEUX,TO HOOGS,DEBB MENDOZA, R

c                        09:50      13:35      11:18     13:50R'M   11:05
                         GRIFFIN, P|                    |WARNER,  M|
                         D&C       |                    |RETINA RET|
                         SEID,ELAIN|                    |CRAVEN,BET|

d                        10:50
                         HOLTON,  J
                         ATRHROPLAS
                         KELLOG,AND

------------------------------------------------------------------------------
WORK/DT:00/00/00       RM:        TM:    BLOCK:     0

  Enter item number:
```

First available   Urology block   Booked Case
time for OR 1   7:30 - 12:00   S U R G E O N
(Green)   (Magenta)   PROCEDURE
                                            PATIENT (Red)

Behind each case is
the ORSOS Data
Record described on
the following pages.

How the SCHEDULER works:

The SCHEDULER replaces the manual scheduling book by automating the appointment function. Inquiries about available time and the booking of cases can be made for individual surgeons, procedures and/or block times. Special checks are performed, eliminating conflicts in bookings between surgeons, surgeon privileges, nursing staff, rooms, special equipment, anesthesia availability and meetings. Only a minimum of case information is needed to book. All changes and/or additional information can be added to the record later. Patient data can be sent and received directly to and from the Admission Office.

On the day before surgery, schedules are printed and distributed throughout the hospital as needed. In addition, the Case Records are printed. Nursing assignments and last minute changes are made by the Charge Nurse using the Real Time Scheduler and these are displayed on the *ORSOS* surgical monitor.

The circulating nurse completes the Case Record information about times, staff activities, delays, etc. After the case is completed, this information is entered into *ORSOS* by clerical personnel. The OR Log is then printed and *ORSOS* prepares and prints the Daily Statistics on the day's volume, utilization and staff productivity.

CASE DATA

Each patient's *ORSOS* record contains many items of data. To simplify and organize the operator's data management effort, patient data items are logically grouped and displayed on six different *ORSOS* screens. Function keys permit the operator to quickly move between the screens in any sequence, displaying the data contained in a patient's record. Full screen editing and "HELP" windows are available.

SUMMARY DATA

```
SUMMARY DATA    CASE NO:    84  PATIENT:  SEID, ELAINE        CHNG
------------------------------------------------------------------
ORSOS CASE NO: 84    (28)PROCEDURE DATE: 10/03/85 (2)START:   09:50
(50)PT.NAME:    SEID, ELAINE              (1)LENGTH:         00:35
(51)PATIENT NO:        (56)BIRTHDATE: 02/01/50SETUP:         00:10
(52)MED REC NO:        (53)SEX:      F        CLEANUP:       00:10
(55)ROOM-BED:          (54)IP/OP        1
(31)SURGEON ID:  A1010       SURG.NAME: GRIFFIN, PHILLIP
(32)ASST.SURG:               ASST.NAME:
(30)ADMIT MD ID: A1010       ADMIT.NAME:
(36)ANEST MD ID: A1005       ANEST NAME:
(60)ANEST TYPE:  1
(61)ANEST AGENT:             (62)COMP.CODE:
(61)OPER RM NO: OR 2            OPER ROOM: OPERATING ROOM #2
(69)PROCEDURE ID:090           PREV. CANCELED:
     D&C
     ADDITIONAL PROCEDURES:
           (71)              (72)            (73)
           (74)              (75)            (76)

(96)CASE COMMENTS:

------------------------------------------------------------------
Enter item number:
```

The Summary Data screen summarizes important data about each case such as the patient's name, procedure, surgeon, room, case length, etc.

ADMITTING DATA

```
ADMITTING DATA  CASE NO:        84  PATIENT:  SEID, ELAINE    CHNG
------------------------------------------------------------------
ORSOS CASE NO:      84          SURGEON:        GRIFFIN, P
PROCEDURE DATE: 12/22/90        PROCEDURE:      D&C
     PT.NAME: SEID, ELAINE  BOOK DATE:   08/27/85
     HOME ADDRESS:              (6)EMPLOYER:MOBILE PAPER SHRED
        (1)STREET:2256 SEAN LANE  (7)STREET:  1085 ORCHARD STREET
        (2)CITY:GRAND JUNCTION    (8)CITY:    GRAND JUNCTION
        (3)STATE:CO (4)ZIP:80103  (9)STATE:CO (10)ZIP: 80127
(5)HOME PHONE:303-349-4967       (11)WORK PHONE:303-544-3895
(12)IN EMERGENCY CONTACT: FRED SEID
(13)RELATIONSHIP: HUSBAND        (23)ADMIT DATE: 10/02/85
(14)PHONE:303-349-3957              PREV.ADMIT DATE:
(15)ANEST TYPE: LOCAL               (24)RELIGION:PROT
(16)INSURANCE CARRIER:AETNA         (25)PT.BDATE:12/22/53
      (17)GROUP#:39475-973          (26)PT. AGE:35
      (18)GROUP#:675749-6456        (27)SMOKES:NO
(19)PRE-CERTIFICATION:  (20)COMPLETED:  (28)TAKEN BY: KB
(21)DIAGNOSIS: INTRAUTERINE HEMORRHAGE
(22)          NOTES:

TESTS ORDERED:  (29):3 (30):   (31):   (32):   (33):    (34):
                (35)   (36)    (37):   (38):   (39):    (40):
------------------------------------------------------------------
Enter item number:
```

The Admitting Data screen captures all data required by the hospital's admitting department.

TIMES AND DATES

```
TIMES & DATES   CASE NO:      84  PATIENT: SEID, ELAINE      CHNG
------------------------------------------------------------------
(2)TIME SCHEDULED TO START:    09:50  (18)START RELIEF ANESTHIO:
(3)TO FOLLOW PREVIOUS CASE:           (19)START 1ST RELIEF SCRUB-1:
(1)ESTIMATED CASE LENGTH:      00:35  (20)START 2ND RELIEF SCRUB-1:
(4)TIME PICK UP FOR SURGERY:   09:18  (21)START 1ST RELIEF SCRUB-2:
(5)TIME ADMIT TO OR SUITE:     09:24  (22)START 2ND RELIEF SCRUB-2:
(6)TIME ENTER OR:              09:45  (23)START 1ST RELIEF CIRC-1:
(7)TIME ANESTHE START:         09:55  (24)START 2ND RELIEF CIRC-1:
(8)TIME OF INCISION:           10:00  (25)START 1ST RELIEF CIRC-2:
(9)TIME OF CLOSURE:            11:33  (26)START 2ND RELIEF CIRC-2:
(10)TIME LEAVE OR:             11:44  (27)PREFERRED START TIME:
(11)TIME ADMIT TO RECVERY:     11:00    TIME CASE BOOKED:    00:35
(12)TIME ANESTHESIA ENDS:      11:55    TIME LAST CHANGED:   03:36
(13)TIME LEAVE RECOVERY:       12:05  (28)DATE OF PROCEDURE: 10/03/85
(14)SPECIAL TIME-1 START:             DATE CASE BOOKED:    09/01/85
(15)SPECIAL TIME-1 STOP:              DATE LAST CHANGED:   10/03/85
(16)SPECIAL TIME-2 START:             (29)DATE PREFERRED:
(17)SPECIAL TIME-2 STOP:

------------------------------------------------------------------
Enter item number:U
```

The Times and Dates screen contains time and information about the case. Times can be collected by surgeon and by procedure

STAFF DATA

```
STAFF          CASE NO: 84    PATIENT:   SEID, ELAINE          CHNG
------------------------------------------------------------------------
(30)ADMITTING DR:                A1010   MACK, STEVE
(31)SURGEON:                     A1010   MACK, STEVE
(32)ASST.SURG-1:
(33)ASST.SURG-2:
(34)ASST.SURG-3:
(35)RESIDENT:
(36)ANESTHES:                    A1005   RAMIREZ, MICHELE
(37)RELIEF ANESTHES:
(38)SCRUB-1:
(39)1ST RELIEF SCRUB-1:          A1012   JOHNSON, JUDY
(40)2ND RELIEF SCRUB-1:          A1003   NESS, ANN
(41)SCRUB-2:
(42)1ST RELIEF SCRUB-2:
(43)2ND RELIEF SCRUB-2:
(44)CIRCULATING-1:
(45)1ST RELIEF CIRC-1:           A1008   NELL, KATE
(46)2ND RELIEF CIRC-1:
(47)CIRCULATING-2:
(48)1ST RELIEF CIRC-2:
(49)2ND RELIEF CIRC-2:
------------------------------------------------------------------------
Enter item number:
```

The Staff Data screen contains the names and positions of all personnel involved in the case.

PATIENT DATA

```
PATIENT DATA     CASE NO:   -84  PATIENT:   SEID, ELAINE      CHNG
------------------------------------------------------------------------
CASE#: 84       (50)PT.NAME: SEID, ELAINE
     (51)PAT #:              (52)MED REC#:        (53)SEX: 2
(54)IP/OP:1  (55)ROOM/BED:       (56)BIRTHDATE:02/01/50  (57)MAJ/MIN: 2
(58)DRG#: 0  (59)TYPE OF CASE: 2(60)ANESTHETIC TECH:1  (61)OP RM: OR2

USER DEFINED STAFF          (62)1:  (63)2:       (64)3:
USER'S ALPH/NUM     (65)1:  (66)2:  (67)3:       (68)4:
(70)WOUND CLASSIFICATION:  3    (71)TISSUE/SPECIMEN SENT:

PROCEDURES:
     (72)  090      D&C     (76)
     (73)                   (77)
     (74)                   (78)
     (75)

OP SITES: (79) 62    (80) 0  (81) 0  (82) 0  (83) 0  (84)   0

(95)UNITS BLOOD RESERVED:
(93)REASON FOR DELAY: 2 (94)DISPOSITION: 1 (96)UNITS BLOOD USED:
(97)CASE COMMENTS NEXT LINE:            (98)       (99)

------------------------------------------------------------------------
Enter item number:
```

The Patient Data screen contains specific patient related data such as medical record number, wound classification, operative sites, and user defined data elements.

RESOURCES DATA

```
CASE RESOURCES    CASE NO:    84  PATIENT:   SEID, ELAINE     CHNG
------------------------------------------------------------------------
RESOURCE ID          DESCRIPTION
(83)    A1006            INTRAUTERINE SUCTION
(84)
(85)
(86)
(87)
(88)
(89)
(90)
(91)

ADDITIONAL COMPLICATIONS:

(93)

(94)


------------------------------------------------------------------------
Enter item number:
```

The Case Resources screen contains the major equipment used for the case such as C-Arm, Microscopes, etc.

SURGERY SCHEDULES

ORSOS prepares two versions of the daily OR schedule. A long form of the schedule, designed to be used by the OR staff, lists cases within rooms. A condensed "short" schedule is also available for distribution to nursing units, admitting, ancillary departments, and other need-to-know areas.

Schedule formats can be customized by each user and schedules can be electronically passed to your HIS for display around the hospital.

CASE LOGS

The Daily OR Log details all case activity. As with the Short and Long schedules, the *ORSOS* system provides a variety of formats from which to choose.

CASE RECORD SHEET

A preprinted form has been designed to accommodate all of the data stored on each case and to provide space for additional information recorded during the case. This information can be handwritten in the lower portion of the CASE RECORD SHEET if it is data to be entered by the operator following the case. (Data entered prior to surgery is printed on the sheet before the case, saving duplicate effort on the part of the nursing staff.)

The upper portion of the CASE RECORD SHEET includes nursing information which is not part of the patient's *ORSOS* record. The CASE RECORD SHEET may replace the hospital's current intraoperative notes, if desired.

SCHEDULER Benefits:

- ➤ *Eliminates potential conflicts in the schedule between surgeons, surgeon privileges, nursing staff, rooms, and special equipment.*
- ➤ *Fully supports first-come-first-served, block and modified block scheduling practices.Provides fast, on-line "lookup" of vital scheduling information.*
- ➤ *Prints schedules for any day's cases on demand.*
- ➤ *Provides unlimited comments about each case including "type-over" procedure descriptions and assignment of multiple surgeons to a case.*
- ➤ *Provides the schedule in either a short form, containing data of interest to nursing units, admitting office and other hospital departments, or a long form, designed for use within the operating suite.*
- ➤ *Provides a CASE RECORD SHEET with all currently available data printed for that case which is completed during the case.*
- ➤ *Automates the formal OR LOG which is often maintained manually by the department.Calculates daily statistics concerning volumes, utilization and productivity.*
- ➤ *Provides surgeons and management with the confidence that all the hospital's resources necessary for a case will be available as scheduled.*

➼ *Provides a dynamic real-time scheduling aid for the Charge Nurse in directing the department's activity.*

➼ *Integrates directly into the hospital's Admission, Discharge and Transfer computer system to share patient demographic data, eliminating redundant data input.*

INVENTORY

INVENTORY:

- Maintains the **Preference Cards for each surgeon** with the preferred equipment and supplies associated with each procedure.

- Prints the **Preference Cards for a day's cases** on demand. Provides full inventory control capabilities in determining stock on hand, stock needing re-ordering, and re-order quantity. It fully supports Case Cart systems.

- Maintains complete **Vendor Profiles** for each of your suppliers.

- Prints **Patient Charges**.

- Tracks **Implant Usage** and produces Implant Log.

- Provides inventory **Cost Accounting** including breakouts between labor and supply costs by procedure, and comparisons between individual surgeon costs.

INVENTORY FUNCTION MENU

```
        (1)     HOSPITAL PREFERENCE CARDS
        (2)     SURGEON PREFERENCE CARDS
        (3)     INVENTORY MAINTENANCE
        (4)     VENDOR MAINTENANCE
        (5)     TRAY MAINTENANCE
        (6)     ACTUAL USAGE UPDATE
        (7)     SUPPLY REQUISITIONS
        (8)     INVENTORY RECEIVING
        (9)     IMPLANT MAINTENANCE


        (10)    INVENTORY REPORTS


Enter item number:
```

How INVENTORY works:

On the day before surgery, the Preference Cards are printed for each case scheduled. The equipment and supplies are readied. After each case is completed, the patient's record is updated with any supplies used that were not on the preference card. The Patient Charges are then printed automatically and sent to the hospital's financial system. *ORSOS* then updates the inventory levels for each supply item, determines which items need re-ordering and prints Supply requisitions. When supplies are received, the inventory levels are adjusted and the requisition tracking system updated.

REPORTER

The REPORTER:

- Prepares and prints monthly and year-to-date management reports.
- Links directly with our Report Generator, allowing preparation of customized reports.

REPORTER FUNCTION MENU

```
(1) GENERATE INDIVIDUAL REPORTS
(2) SELECT GROUP REPORTS
(3) RUN GROUP REPORTS
(4) PRINT GROUP REPORTS




Enter item number:
```

At the end of each month, the detailed information collected in the CONTROLLER and SCHEDULER is used to prepare the management reports. The REPORTER automatically prepares and prints reports on demand covering the following areas:

- **VOLUME STATISTICS** on major cases, minor cases, inpatients, outpatients, anesthesia, etc., by surgeon, anesthesiologist, service and unit.
- **UTILIZATION STATISTICS** details room usage by day of week and hour of day. It also includes utilization statistics by surgeon and service. It tracks delayed, run-over and canceled cases by surgeon and service.
- **PRODUCTIVITY STATISTICS** summarizes the department's productivity in both hours and dollars, comparing both fixed and flexed budgets with actual usage.
- **SURGEON TIME PER PROCEDURE** details the historical time each surgeon has been using per procedure performed. This information is used in the SCHEDULER module to estimate case length.
- **BLOCK UTILIZATION** analyzes the usage of block allocations to insure maximum utilization of your facility if you use block scheduling.
- **COST/DRG REPORT** provides analysis of the direct surgical department costs, both labor- and supply-associated withe each procedure, surgeon and DRG category encountered by your department.

THE ORSOS EXPANSION MODULES

ORSOS may be optimized by including these fully integrated expansion modules:

- **PERIOPERATIVE CHARTING** This paperless bedside charting environment uses a high speed network and light pens to do complete patient charting from pre-operative assessment to post-anesthesia recovery.

- **REMOTE SCHEDULING** REMOTE links surgeons' offices to the hospital's O.R. scheduling office to provide input of patient pre-admission data, viewing of surgery times and a summary of all a surgeon's cases or his cases for today.

- **PERSONNEL SCHEDULING** This module provides a completely integrated management information system for position control, scheduling, staffing and productivity/personnel reporting.

- *ORSOS* **Bar Code Option** for Inventory. Bar Coding is fully integrated in the the *ORSOS* Inventory module to provide the user with an efficient means of entering data using bar code readers.

- **The ATLINK HIS Interfaces**

  1. The **ADT** ATLINK accesses the mainframe admitting system for collection of pre-admission data.

  2. The **Charge** ATLINK passes patient charge information to the hospital's financial system.

  3. The **Materials Management** ATLINK uses mainframe inventory data for tracking usage and quantity on hand, generating supply requisitions and much more.

  4. The **Schedules** ATLINK passes *ORSOS* Schedules for display on HIS Terminals.

- **CORPORATE REPORTING** This expansion function allows you to compile management reports across multiple surgery locations within the hospital corporation, plus provide "roll up" reports for all surgery locations.

- **WORD PROCESSING** Access to your favorite word processing program is available at the touch of a key from the *ORSOS* main menu.

REMOTE SCHEDULING

REMOTE SCHEDULING is integrated into the *ORSOS* Scheduler using advanced technology linking surgeons' offices to the hospital's surgery scheduling office. Surgeons may request surgery time, input patient pre-admission data, view a summary of all their cases booked for surgery and view today's surgery schedule for adjusted start times and remarks about their cases. REMOTE SCHEDULING may also be located in the surgeon's lounge or other sites in or outside the hospital, allowing a surgeon easy access to information about the progress of today's OR schedule.

REMOTE SCHEDULING MAIN MENU

```
                  (1) Edit Requests to Schedule
                  (2) ORSOS Return Status
                  (3) View Scheduled Cases
                  (4) View Today's Cases
                  (5)Exit and return to DOS




    Enter item number:
```

How REMOTE SCHEDULING works:

At remote sites (a surgeon's office or the doctor's lounge, etc.) a surgeon or member of the surgeon's office staff may enter a request to schedule a case, change case information or request to cancel a case. Pre-admission information may also be entered by the office staff and sent, with the schedule request, electronically via modem to the hospital scheduling office.

The hospital scheduling office is notified immediately upon receipt of the request and with the assistance of user friendly Help windows, the Scheduler may view the request, book the case and communicate the results back to the surgeon's office. Requests may be batched and handled as time permits or booked immediately upon receipt. Requests that cannot be met (e.g. no available time) can be communicated back to the surgeon's office with suggestions for other dates and times. The surgeon may view the status of all requests and information about a surgeon's cases at any time.

As the day's cases progress, the surgery department charge nurse may quickly input remarks about each case start time such as "delayed 30 minutes" or "moved to Room 3". Today's schedule with the remarks can then be viewed from any remote workstation as well as printed at the surgeon's office.

REMOTE SCHEDULING Benefits:
>> *Remote Scheduling will enhance the quality of service provided to the hospital's surgeons by allowing them easy access to view scheduling information and giving them notice of last minute schedule changes. It will allow them to request cases without encountering "busy phone lines" or being placed on hold.*
>> *Remote Scheduling will improve the management of the scheduling office by allowing the schedulers to book cases as time permits rather than juggle multiple phone calls. It will significantly decrease the time required by the charge nurse to call each office or answer phone inquiries about changes for today's schedule.*

BAR CODING CAPABILITIES

BAR CODING is fully integrated into the *ORSOS* INVENTORY module to provide the *ORSOS* user with an efficient means of entering data. *ORSOS* BAR CODING conforms to all health care bar coding industry standards (HIBC) utilizing Code 39. Equipment consists of both stationary and portable bar code readers integrated into microcomputers on the *ORSOS* network.

ORSOS uses BAR CODING to perform the following functions:

1. Record all supplies used during a case

2. Track the use of and location of instruments, trays and equipment

3. Receive items into the INVENTORY module from the department's suppliers

4. Produce bar code labels for all surgery supplies

5. Record the department's physical inventory

6. Speed the building and revision of surgeon preference cards

How BAR CODING works:

When supplies are received from the department's suppliers, *ORSOS* BAR CODING allows the user to wand in the item's bar code and the quantity received, automatically updating the *ORSOS* INVENTORY quantity on hand for the product. Simultaneously, bar code labels can be generated for specific items if required.

During the case, bar code labels are removed from the packaging and affixed to the charge capture document. During the *ORSOS* post case data input, the supplies used, represented by the barcode labels, are then quickly scanned into *ORSOS*. The quantities on hand are automatically adjusted and charges are generated.

To aid the Central Supply staff in maintaining inventory for instruments, trays and equipment, *ORSOS* BAR CODING provides the user with the ability to wand items with their destination as they enter and leave the department. By tracking capital equipment in this matter, Central Supply knows the location and status of capital equipment and each instrument tray and at all times.

Complete physical inventories are taken periodically using hand-held wands, by moving through the department supply storage areas and scanning in items and quantities. The contents of the hand-held wands are automatically read by *ORSOS*, and quantity on hand figures are adjusted to reflect newly reconciled information.

ORSOS BAR CODING is also incorporated into building preference cards to speed their development. Users simply bar code supplies and equipment requested by the surgeon, and *ORSOS* builds the preference card.

BENEFITS
- ➻ *Provides an easy-to-use means of inputting vital inventory information.*
- ➻ *The time required to reconcile the physical inventory to the system inventory is greatly reduced.*
- ➻ *Maximum savings are realized through enhanced inventory control.*
- ➻ *Improves tracking of trays and equipment*
- ➻ *Increases surgeon satisfaction.*
- ➻ *Integrates with hospital-wide materials management practices.*

HARDWARE REQUIREMENTS

ORSOS runs on a local area network. The system is designed to allow workstations to continue processing even in the unlikely event the network encounters problems.

An example of the equipment required is given below.

FILE SERVER

- IBM PS/2 Model 70, l2OMb Hard Disk, 3Mb RAM
- IBM Monochrome Monitor
- IBM DOS VER. 3 .3
- Uninterruptable Power Supply (Elgar 560)

WORKSTATION

- IBM PS/2 Model 30 286, 2OMb Hard Disk, 1 Mb RAM
- IBM Color Monitor (8512) Surge Protector
- IBM DOS VER 3.3
- Tape Backup Unit, External (Mountain Model 60)

NETWORK REQUIREMENTS

- Network Adaptor Cards (any type topology, e.g. Ethernet, Token Ring or Arcnet)
- Novell Advanced Netware Ver. 2 .15 PS/2
- Cable

PRINTER

- HP Laserjet

EXPANSION MODULE COMPONENTS

- IBM Mouse (for Perioperative Charting module)
- Bar code reader with software (for Bar Code module)

Appendix E
The Market Planner®

The Market Planner® Evaluates Your Market and Estimates Market Share!

The analytic and graphic capabilities of The Market Planner enable you to profile your market using any of the demographic, patient, or physician variables in your databases. This information can be clearly displayed in tabular, map and graph formats.

For example, you might want to gain insight into the geographic areas from which patients come by various classifications such as DRG's, product lines, admitting physician or payor. Figures 1, 2, 3 and 4 illustrate tables, maps and graphs which **The Market Planner** is capable of producing to assist in this analysis. Figure 1 indicates the number of HMO patient admissions by zip code and product line. Figure 2 displays where the O.B. patients live to identify potential locations for physician offices. Figure 3 demonstrates the ability of **The Market Planner** to aggregate payor data of hospital patients into key market areas that describe payor mix penetration patterns. Figure 4 is a pie chart of the percentage of HMO patients coming from particular market areas.

Another important use of **The Market Planner** is to determine your market share by DRG or product line by zip code or market areas. This is estimated using data from several of your databases:

- Inpatient discharge file which provides you with the number of admissions by DRG, age, and sex for each geographic area.
- Use rate model for your area which projects admission rates for each geographic area.
- Demographic data which show the number of people in each area by age and sex.
- Map file.

By incorporating assumptions about future hospital utilization, you can calculate both current and projected market share by DRG or product line.

Source: Reprinted with the permission of The Sachs Group Ltd., Evanston, Illinois.

ADMISSIONS OF HMO MEMBERS (BY ZIP CODE AND PRODUCT)

	CARD	OB	ONC	ORTHO	TOTAL
63001	0	0	0	0	0
63011	29	74	14	38	155
63017	49	60	21	51	181
63018	0	1	0	0	1
63021	22	80	6	19	127
63022	0	1	0	0	1
63025	2	5	0	7	14
63026	2	15	1	11	29
63031	7	28	3	8	46
63032	0	0	0	1	1
63033	3	35	4	7	49
63034	2	3	2	1	8
63038	0	7	1	4	12
63040	0	0	0	1	1
63042	3	7	5	5	20
63043	6	17	2	6	31
63044	3	13	1	3	20
63074	0	3	5	2	10
63088	0	5	3	3	11
63105	3	7	1	7	18
63114	6	28	4	10	48
63117	4	2	1	3	10
63119	5	17	9	20	51
63121	2	6	1	3	12
63122	11	27	1	13	52
TOTAL	159	441	85	223	908

FIG. 1

Figures 5, 6, 7 and 8 illustrate such market share data for cardiology using **The Market Planner's** table, map and bar chart capabilities.

Product line, market areas, payor groups, physician groups can all be defined, modified and changed rapidly to examine relationships and spot new opportunities.

The Market Planner® Projects Changes in Admissions/Patient Days!

One of the most valuable uses of **The Market Planner** is the projection of changes in admissions or patient days over time both for your market area as a whole and for your institution specifically. This is accomplished using projections of changes in the size and characteristics of the population of your market areas together with use rate models and market share estimates. Patient discharge data are employed to provide a historical basis for your hospital's experience. Use rate models are based on national, regional or local inpatient hospital discharge statistics.

The projection capabilities are extremely flexible and allow you to alter various assumptions to fit your hospital and market place. For example, you

ADMISSIONS OF OBSTETRICS PATIENTS

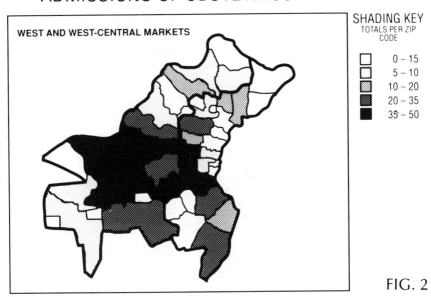

FIG. 2

ADMISSIONS OF HMO MEMBERS BY MARKET

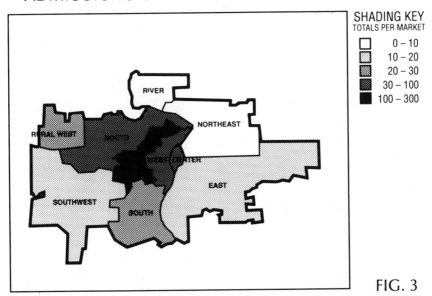

FIG. 3

PERCENT OF ADMISSIONS OF HMO MEMBERS BY MARKET

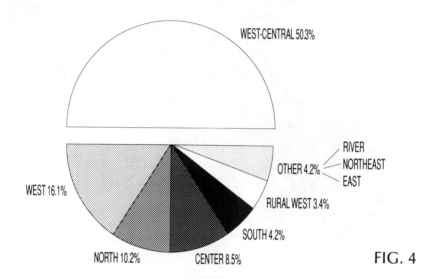

WEST-CENTRAL 50.3%

OTHER 4.2% — RIVER / NORTHEAST / EAST

WEST 16.1%

RURAL WEST 3.4%

SOUTH 4.2%

NORTH 10.2%   CENTER 8.5%   FIG. 4

MIDWEST HOSPITAL
MARKET SHARE AND UTILIZATION PROJECTION
For Market: WEST

Product Line	Market Share (x100)			Expected Market Size		
	1987	1992	Change	1987	1992	% Chg.
UNCLASSIFIED	0.00	0.00	0.00	58	57	−2.62
CARDIOLOGY	2.41	2.54	0.13	11,775	12,282	4.31
CATCH ALL	4.19	4.46	0.27	1,240	1,283	3.44
GENERAL SURGERY	3.27	3.51	0.24	7,279	7,448	2.33
GYNECOLOGY	5.15	5.58	0.43	3,571	3,628	1.59
INTERNAL MEDICINE	2.27	2.41	0.15	12,884	13,302	3.24
MEDICAL SUBSPEC.	2.62	2.78	0.17	8,795	9,090	3.35
NEURO/PSYCH/SUB. AB.	1.65	1.77	0.12	8,357	8,574	2.60
NEUROSURGERY	1.25	1.34	0.09	963	986	2.32
NEWBORN	5.30	5.86	0.56	8,490	8,442	−0.57
OBSTETRICS	4.49	5.55	1.05	11,308	10,077	−10.89
ONCOLOGY	3.36	3.61	0.25	4,344	4,447	2.38
OPHTHALMOLOGY	1.69	1.80	0.11	1,180	1,219	3.32
ORTHOPEDICS	3.85	4.13	0.28	9,033	9,259	2.51
OTOLARYNGOLOGY	3.37	3.78	0.41	2,256	2,214	−1.89
PEDIATRICS	0.11	0.12	0.01	3,626	3,555	−1.98
PLASTIC SURGERY	1.88	2.05	0.17	1,063	1,073	0.89
SURGICAL SUBSPEC.	1.80	1.97	0.17	2,225	2,236	0.52
UROLOGY	1.85	1.96	0.11	5,086	5,268	3.58
TOTAL	3.03	3.30	0.27	103,535	104,441	0.87

NOTE: UNCLASSIFIED IS ALL ADMISSIONS WITH MISSING DISCHARGE DRGS OR ICD9S   FIG. 5

CARDIOLOGY PATIENT ORIGIN BY ZIP CODE

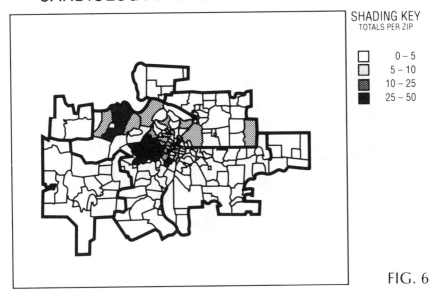

SHADING KEY
TOTALS PER ZIP

☐   0 – 5
▦   5 – 10
▩   10 – 25
■   25 – 50

FIG. 6

CARDIOLOGY SHARE BY MARKET – 1988

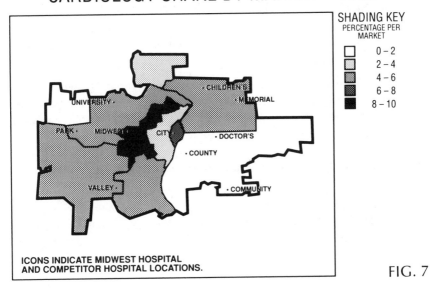

SHADING KEY
PERCENTAGE PER
MARKET

☐   0 – 2
▦   2 – 4
▩   4 – 6
▨   6 – 8
■   8 – 10

ICONS INDICATE MIDWEST HOSPITAL
AND COMPETITOR HOSPITAL LOCATIONS.

FIG. 7

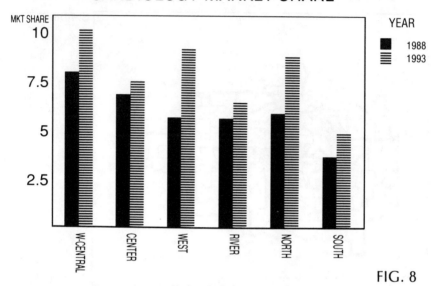

CARDIOLOGY MARKET SHARE

FIG. 8

may wish to alter the use rates to reflect anticipated shifts to outpatient facilities for specific DRG's or product lines. Other assumptions that can be altered include:

- Mean length of stay for each product line and market.
- Changes in market share anticipated as a result of planned product modifications, promotional activity, closures of hospitals and contracting strategies.

Figure 9 illustrates current vs. projected admissions and patient days by product line for a specific hospital. Figure 10 displays in map form projected admissions for obstetrics for each market area. Figure 11 displays in map form total projected admissions for cardiology for each market area.

The Market Planner® Targets Opportunities For Growth!

The results of projections of change in the underlying demographics of your market areas will suggest opportunities for product targeting. For example, projected increases in the elderly population may suggest opportunities for certain specialties such as cardiology, orthopedics or ophthalmology. Furthermore, entirely new services may be suggested, such as retirement living facilities.

ADMISSIONS AND PATIENT DAYS PROJECTION
MIDWEST HOSPITAL
For Market: WEST

Product Line	In-Patient Admissions			In-Patient Days		
	1987	1992	% Chg.	1987	1992	% Chg.
UNCLASSIFIED	0	0	0.00	0	0	0.00
CARDIOLOGY	284	296	4.31	2,952	3,079	4.31
CATCH ALL	52	54	3.44	654	676	3.44
GENERAL SURGERY	238	244	2.33	2,142	2,192	2.33
GYNECOLOGY	184	187	1.59	986	1,002	1.59
INTERNAL MEDICINE	292	301	3.24	2,122	2,191	3.24
MEDICAL SUBSPEC.	230	238	3.35	1,542	1,594	3.35
NEURO/PSYCH/SUB. AB.	138	142	2.60	1,260	1,293	2.60
NEUROSURGERY	12	12	2.32	204	209	2.32
NEWBORN	450	447	−0.57	1,752	1,742	−0.57
OBSTETRICS	508	453	−10.89	1,844	1,643	−10.89
ONCOLOGY	146	149	2.38	798	817	2.38
OPHTHALMOLOGY	20	21	3.32	96	99	3.32
ORTHOPEDICS	348	357	2.51	2,880	2,952	2.51
OTOLARYNGOLOGY	76	75	−1.89	86	84	−1.89
PEDIATRICS	4	4	−1.98	12	12	−1.98
PLASTIC SURGERY	20	20	0.89	134	135	0.89
SURGICAL SUBSPEC.	40	40	0.52	682	686	0.52
UROLOGY	94	97	3.58	526	545	3.58
TOTAL	3,136	3,137	0.03	20,672	20,951	1.35

NOTE: UNCLASSIFIED IS ALL ADMISSIONS WITH MISSING DISCHARGE DRGS OR ICD9S

FIG. 9

PROJECTED OBSTETRICS ADMISSIONS – 1993

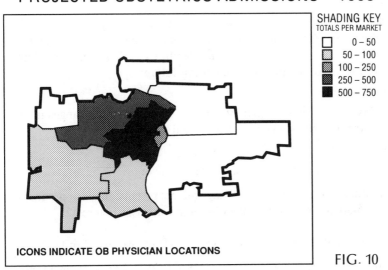

SHADING KEY
TOTALS PER MARKET

- 0 – 50
- 50 – 100
- 100 – 250
- 250 – 500
- 500 – 750

ICONS INDICATE OB PHYSICIAN LOCATIONS

FIG. 10

PROJECTED CARDIOLOGY ADMISSIONS – 1993

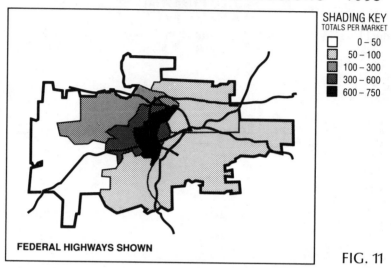

SHADING KEY
TOTALS PER MARKET

☐   0 – 50
▨ 50 – 100
▦ 100 – 300
▩ 300 – 600
■ 600 – 750

FEDERAL HIGHWAYS SHOWN

FIG. 11

The **Market Planner** allows you to enhance this opportunity analysis by integrating utilization projections with financial data. It takes the forecasted admissions/patient days and computes DRG or product line specific net revenue forecasts using charge and cost data from your institution. If historical charge or cost data are not available, estimates for the projection may be used.

The results of this analysis will suggest opportune products as well as potential problem areas which may require additional marketing attention or revision of the hospital's strategy. The flexibility of **The Market Planner** allows you to make assumptions regarding future:

- Payor mix
- Revenue by product line by payor (e.g., anticipated changes in reimbursement by Medicare, HMO's and other payor groups)
- Inflation
- Changes in costs by product line by payor

An illustration of projected changes in net revenue for each product line across all market areas is displayed in table format in Figure 12.

Increase Market Share—Grow Revenue—Improve Profitability

Developed and marketed by **THE SACHS GROUP, The Market Planner**® is the advanced software system designed to help you achieve your strategic

COST AND REVENUE PROJECTION
MIDWEST HOSPITAL
For Payor Group: TOTAL

Product Line	Costs		Revenues		Revenues–Costs	
	1987	1992	1987	1992	1987	1992
UNCLASSIFIED	$67	$74	$53	$58	–$15	–$16
CARDIOLOGY	$13,657	$15,023	$20,556	$22,612	$6,899	$7,589
CATCH ALL	$2,522	$2,774	$2,607	$2,868	$85	$94
GENERAL SURGERY	$7,148	$7,863	$9,356	$10,291	$2,208	$2,429
GYNECOLOGY	$3,947	$4,342	$4,464	$4,911	$517	$569
INTERNAL MEDICI	$7,051	$7,756	$8,364	$9,201	$1,314	$1,445
MEDICAL SUBSPEC	$3,800	$4,180	$4,706	$5,177	$906	$997
NEURO/PSYCH/SUB	$3,550	$3,905	$5,210	$5,731	$1,660	$1,826
NEUROSURGERY	$1,632	$1,795	$2,037	$2,240	$405	$445
NEWBORN	$2,381	$2,619	$2,412	$2,653	$31	$34
OBSTETRICS	$6,071	$6,679	$7,030	$7,733	$959	$1,055
ONCOLOGY	$3,392	$3,731	$4,966	$5,463	$1,574	$1,732
OPHTHALMOLOGY	$130	$142	$196	$216	$67	$74
ORTHOPEDICS	$13,374	$14,712	$16,806	$18,487	$3,432	$3,775
OTOLARYNGOLOGY	$621	$683	$738	$812	$117	$129
PEDIATRICS	$85	$93	$119	$131	$35	$38
PLASTIC SURGERY	$580	$638	$541	$596	–$39	–$43
SURGICAL SUBSPE	$1,760	$1,936	$2,510	$2,761	$750	$825
UROLOGY	$3,108	$3,419	$4,066	$4,473	$958	$1,054
Total	$74,876	$82,363	$96,740	$106,414	$21,864	$24,050

NOTE: UNCLASSIFIED IS ALL ADMISSIONS WITH MISSING DISCHARGE DRGS
NOTE: AMOUNTS ARE DOLLARS IN THOUSANDS   FIG. 12

objectives. **The Market Planner** works with databases specific to your institution and market. The comprehensive modeling, analysis, mapping and graphing features of **The Market Planner**:

- Evaluate the nature of your market and estimate your market share by DRG or product line for each market area.
- Project changes in the marketplace and estimate resulting changes in admissions and patient days at your hospital.
- Target opportunities for growth by integrating market-driven utilization and financial projections.

The Market Planner contains information specific to your market and hospital:

- Demographic data from the 1980 census, current year estimates, and five year projections of the population in your market areas as you define them. Data are normally provided at the zip code level, but optionally can be supplied at the census tract or block group level. The data include age, income, sex, housing, education and other census information.

- Inpatient hospitalization rates by DRG, ICD9-CM code, age and sex for all census regions. Customized local use rates can be developed where area-specific patient origin databases exist.

- Data from your institution's patient record file containing patient information such as DRG, ICD9-CM code, charges, admitting, attending or referring physician, length of stay, zip code, age, sex, payor, etc. Variables contained in the databases are limited only by the availability of information and file storage capacity.

- Medical staff database containing practice information such as office location, specialty, age, board certification, group affiliation, etc.

- Cartographic database for creating maps of your market areas as you have defined them.

- Competitor databases such as hospital and non-hospital facilities and utilization, area physicians, HMO's, etc. to establish the hospitals' competitive position.

THE SACHS GROUPS
Advanced Systems For Planning And Marketing

Appendix F
The Physician Practice Planner ™

The Physician Practice Planner™ is designed to help you increase revenue through development of enhanced physician/patient activity. The Physician Practice Planner™ is an extension of THE MARKET PLANNER,® the software core of THE SACHS PLAN.^{SM}

The Physician Practice Planner links demographic information about your market with the best and most current data available to...

- forecast office visits by market segment and physician specialty
- identify over- and under-served areas by comparing physician supply with demand
- estimate expected follow-up care related to visit volumes

The Physician Practice Planner is essential for expanding revenue through physician development and placement. It enables you to design and analyze strategies for...

- physician placement
- expansion of existing practices
- acquisition of new practices

The Physician Practice Planner allows you to care for your most important customer...the physician.

Applications include:

- Controlling assumptions regarding physician visit rates and productivity by specialty
- Estimating visit volumes by physician specialty and market
- Identifying physician need and supply by specialty and market
- Documenting expected demand for new physician offices in existing market areas
- Researching the loyalty of doctors to your hospital
- Estimating follow-up care by specialty (e.g., hospital admissions, ambulatory surgery, return office visits, referrals, ancillary usage, etc.)

Source: Reprinted with the permission of The Sachs Group Ltd., Evanston, Illinois.

Output includes:

- Converting findings into tables/reports, maps or graphs
- Producing standard reports of five year forecasts:

  Visit Projection Tables store both expected office visits and office visit rates by visit attribute, physician specialty and market. Visit attributes include: reason for visit, principal diagnosis, disposition of visit, principal payor, lab test indicator, non-medical therapy, X-ray or EKG indicator.

  Visit Need Tables store physician productivity rates, physician supply, numbers of expected physician office visits and estimated/projected physician need by specialty and market.

- Estimating visit volumes by physician specialty and market
- Placing visits by physician specialty and market
- Charting non-medical therapies, follow-up to visits by physician specialty and market
- Mapping physician visit volumes and physician undersupply by physician specialty and market
- Graphing disposition of visits by physician specialty and market

THE SACHS PLAN integrates software, data, education, and support to give you an innovative path for growth. It provides a predictable environment for you to improve your day-to-day strategic decisions.

THE SACHS PLAN is designed by THE SACHS GROUP, a unique gathering of individuals, who understand the needs of your business. The company has established a positive track record with leading institutions throughout the country. THE SACHS GROUP has the intellect, the experience, and the explosive drive to help you respond to the marketplace.

OB OFFICE LOCATIONS — KEY MARKET AREAS

ABSOLUTE POPULATION GROWTH '87—92 — WOMEN AGE 14—44

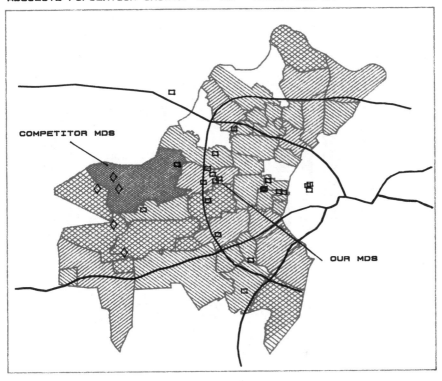

SHADING KEY

BY ZIP CODE

☐	−500− −250
▨	−250− 0
▧	0− 250
▨	250− 500
■	500− 750

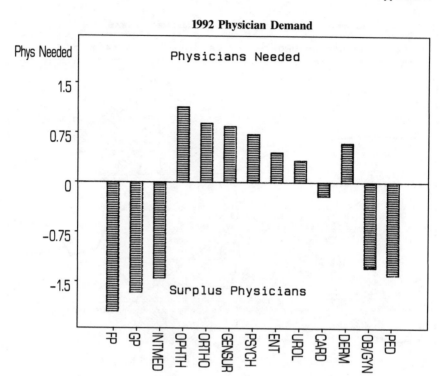

Appendix G
Trendstar Marketing Systems Library

Marketing and Planning with MSL

Determine how best to deploy your marketing resources with Marketing Systems Library (MSL), HBO & Company's new marketing and planning software. MSL complements HBO's other decision support systems by integrating the internal data stored in case mix, cost accounting and departmental systems with data about the external environment. The result: easy access to consistent, accurate and timely information about prices, products, physicians, patient volumes, costs and more.

Why you need MSL

No other market planning system offers strategic planners and marketers the broad range of benefits that HBO & Company's MSL offers. With MSL, you can

- **Identify marketing opportunities.**
  Understand a market's potential in terms of population distribution, socioeconomic characteristics and underlying demand for services. You can then target specific market segments according to expected contribution margin, growth potential, and organizational and community objectives.

- **Optimize the mix of clinical specialties.**
  Assess your physicians in terms of case and payor mix, market penetration, referral networks and practice patterns. MSL will tell you which markets are saturated by given specialties where additional physicians can best be supported.

- **Enhance market share through effective contracting.**
  When you go to the negotiating table, leverage your knowledge of cost behavior, treatment patterns and carrier subscriber volumes. MSL lets you manipulate price reductions and volume increases to negotiate profitable contracts with self-insured employers and other payors.

- **Improve the accuracy of demand forecasts.**
  Increase your confidence in long-range plans and budget projections

---

by using MSL's accurate forecasting tools. The system supports extrapolative, historical-based models as well as demand models based on national and regional draw rates and usage.

- **Know the impact of your decisions before you make them.**
Use MSL simulation capabilities to understand the short and long-term consequences of your marketing decisions based on varying assumptions of reimbursement methods, case mixes, wage and salary indices and market demands.

The Power of MSL

MSL has three primary components that enhance the activities of healthcare marketing and planning professionals: powerful analytic tools, comprehensive databases and presentation-quality color graphics for reporting.

Analysis tools

MSL offers unique views of your clinical, financial and competitive data, giving you valuable insights into healthcare markets.

- **Product line management.**
With MSL, you can optimize your product mix and volume, determine market penetration and the effects of new products, match clinical services with market demand, and monitor the impact of your advertising and promotional campaigns.

- **Demand forecasting.**
Using historical trends or market statistics, MSL can produce forecasts based on product volumes, competitive activity, physician admissions, changes in market share and any number of other data elements.

- **Physician analysis.**
With high quality color maps and graphics, MSL can show physician resource utilization and profitability patterns, practice and referral networks, saturated and underserved markets, and medical staff composition by age, sex, specialty, practice type and location.

- **Payor analysis.**
You can use MSL to analyze the profitability, case mix intensity, geographic concentration and subscriber demographics of each payor. You can also model the impact of reimbursement methodologies on a *pro forma* basis.

- **Competitor analysis.**
MSL also looks at your competitors' market share and spheres of influence, analyzing their product offerings and volumes, admission

trends, productivity comparisons, ancillary service volumes and quality assessments.

Comprehensive data

The comprehensive and precise reporting offered by MSL is your key to accurately defining the healthcare market in which you compete. MSL uses five primary types of data:

- **Case mix and patient detail.**
  MSL uses data from HBO's Case Mix Library and Clinical Cost Accounting systems, which detail clinical, financial and patient origin information.

- **Physician communities.**
  MSL details demographic and geographic information about both admitting and nonadmitting physicians in the hospital's service area. It also tracks medical staff practice patterns, including admissions, resource utilization, product mix and severity, case profitability and referral relationships.

- **Payors and major employers.**
  MSL analyzes payor reimbursement mechanisms, resource consumption, patient severity, subscriber proximity, and inpatient and outpatient product mix. Employers are tracked by location, number of employees and health insurance provided.

- **Population demographics and psychographics.**
  MSL incorporates 1980 census data, current year estimates and future year projections yielding vital population statistics concerning socioeconomic characteristics and lifestyle segmentation. The data can be summarized by county, zip code and census tract.

- **Competing facilities.**
  MSL can profile the services, beds, FTEs, patient days, outpatient and ER visits, and occupancies of your competing facilities. Where state comparative databases are available, you can also evaluate competitors' products, resource utilization, payor mix and mortality rates. And MSL provides nonhospital competitive data for managed care programs, ambulatory care centers and group practices.

Presentation-quality maps

MSL offers two broad categories of crisp, clear color graphics for both problem solving and formal presentation:

Computer-generated maps, with boundary definitions ranging from state, county, zip and census tracts to highways and local streets. You can define your own mapping scales, pinpoint site locations and enter additional map data such trade areas. Sixteen colors are available, and a zoom feature lets you highlight selected areas.

Business graphics, including all standard pie, bar and line charts illustrated on a 16-color printer, in either draft or presentation quality.

Authorized Digital distributor

MSL runs on MicroVAX minicomputers from Digital Equipment Corporation, the world's leading manufacturer of interactive computers. HBO is an Authorized Digital Distributor.

Depend on HBO

HBO's regional representatives and corporate support staff are available to answer questions and provide training in the use of MSL. Let an HBO account representative help you analyze your marketing position and explain more about how MSL can benefit your organization.

CORPORATE HEADQUARTERS
301 Perimeter Center North
Atlanta, Georgia 30346
404-393-6000

Appendix H
Demonstrating Quality of Clinical Outcomes: A Powerful Tool for Market Differentiation

A Case Study

Community Hospital, a 260 bed acute care facility, is interested in increasing volume in its 23 bed obstetric unit, which has been averaging 50% occupancy. The hospital's marketing department has recommended a strategy based on a preferred provider relationship with a local HMO, Patriot Health Plan.

The hospital would leverage its position by focusing on the variables of highest concern to the HMO—Price and Utilization. Community would offer to lower both the per diem, and average length of stay, while improving overall quality. This would greatly increase the "value" of the obstetric services Community provided, enhancing its competitive position. In exchange, the HMO would guarantee a substantial increase in the OB cases directed to Community. The offer would include the following points:

- Lower the percentage of Cesarean Deliveries by 13%, decreasing the payor's average length of stay.
- Reduce the per diem payment by 6.7% from $750 per day to $700.
- PHP would increase Community's obstetric case volume from 190 annual cases to 500 cases.

The combined impact of these changes would result in an average savings of $282 per case to Patriot Health Plan, and an increase of $278,000 to the hospital's bottom line.

The proposal is based on the following market analysis.

Source: Paper presented by Charles M. Jacobs, Chairman, MediQual Systems, Inc., at the Tenth Annual Meeting of the Society for Healthcare Planning and Marketing, May 1–3, 1988. Reprinted with the permission of HBO & Company and MediQual Systems, Inc.

Exhibit 1

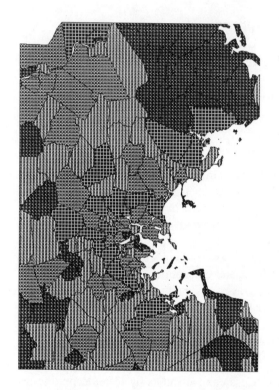

0 –	2258
2259 –	5733
5734 –	8811
8812 –	19884

GREATER METROPOLITAN
BOSTON

POPULATION DISTRIBUTION
BY ZIP CODE
FEMALES 15 – 44
(1987 EST.)

THE COMMUNITY HOSPITAL
PRIMARY SERVICE AREA

- In 1987, Community Hospital's primary service area contains high concentrations of females of childbearing age.

- There has been continued growth in the 15–44 age population due to a strong local economy. (See population trends in Exhibit 2.)

Exhibit 2

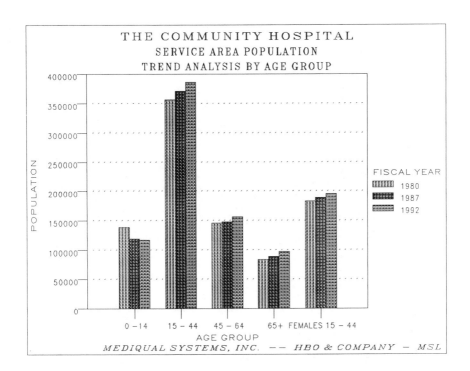

Population trends indicate:

• Pediatric population is declining steadily.

• 15–44 age group is fastest growing segment.

• 45–64 age group is increasing slightly.

• Elderly population is gradually increasing.

• Females from 15 to 44 are increasing at a steady rate, out pacing the overall growth in the population.

Exhibit 3

The Community Hospital: Projected Number of Obstetric Cases in Service Area

Age Group (Female)	Projected Population		Use Rates*		Number of OB Cases		
					Actual	Projected	
	1987	1992	1987	1992	1986	1987	1992
15–19	29,533	25,411	33.0	29.0	1,011	975	737
20–24	37,084	33,897	76.2	70.2	2,824	2,826	2,380
25–29	35,287	34,530	91.2	98.8	3,292	3,218	3,412
30–34	39,518	44,775	57.0	64.0	1,889	2,253	2,866
35–44	57,033	65,037	11.6	13.1	515	662	852
Total	198,455	203,650			9,541	9,934	10,247

*Births/1000 women.

- Population projections indicate that females over the age of 30 are increasing, while those under 30 are decreasing.
- Use rates are expected to increase for women age 25 and over due to the "Baby Boom" generation having children at a later age.
- The overall number of obstetrics cases in the service area are projected to increase over the next five years.

Exhibit 4

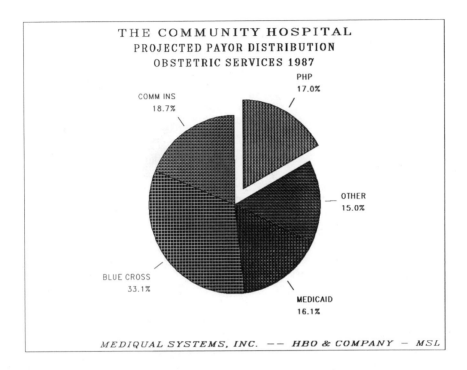

THE COMMUNITY HOSPITAL
PROJECTED PAYOR DISTRIBUTION
OBSTETRIC SERVICES 1987

PHP
17.0%

COMM INS
18.7%

OTHER
15.0%

BLUE CROSS
33.1%

MEDICAID
16.1%

MEDIQUAL SYSTEMS, INC. — — HBO & COMPANY — MSL

- In 1987 PHP represented 17% of Community's obstetric business (190 cases). Reimbursement was based on a per diem.

- Blue Cross and Commercial Insurance represented the largest and most lucrative market segment, reimbursing the hospital based on a discount from charges.

- Medicaid is a less desirable population due to lower reimbursement per case.

Exhibit 5

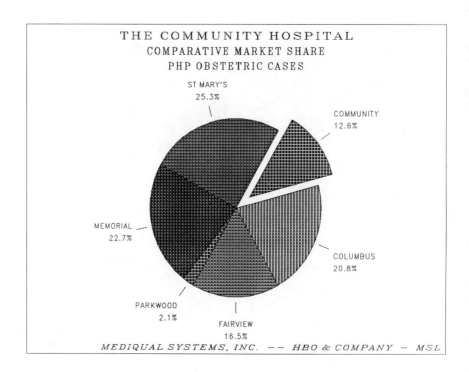

- Community Hospital currently admits 12.6% of PHP's total obstetrics cases (1,508 annual cases).

- St. Mary's, Columbus and Memorial Hospitals each have a larger penetration of PHP's obstetrics market. This is due partly to area demographics (large Catholic population favoring St. Mary's) and the proximity of Memorial and Columbus to areas with higher concentrations of PHP subscribers.

- The demographics of PHP subscribers favor higher income and education levels. While OB cases tend to be less profitable compared to other healthcare services, OB can be used as a "Loss Leader" to ensure other PHP business.

Exhibit 6

Each medical record associated with a surgical procedure should contain evidence of clinical findings which are indications for the procedure. This "Validating" evidence should be based on objective information. If enough validating criteria is collected, a standard can be developed for comparative purposes.

- C-Section validation can be reviewed according to clinical findings of mother and child.

- The MedisGroups standard for "No Findings" cases is between 33% and 51%. This is +1 standard deviation around the MedisGroups mean of 42% (42% if C-Sections have no evidence of clinical validation).

Procedure Validation
Cesarean Section Delivery

Low Validation

- History of Previous C-Section

Medium Validation

- Diastolic Blood Pressure > 120
- Late Deceleration/Loss of Variability
- Fetal Scalp Sample pH <7.25
- Placenta Abruption / Previa
- Prolapsed Cord
- Other Breech
- Diastolic BP > 90 AND Urine Protein > 300 mg
- Labor Arrest

Comparative "No Findings" Range—33% to 51%
Range reflects the mean +1 standard deviation

MEDIQUAL SYSTEMS, INC. -- HBO & COMPANY - MSL

Exhibit 7

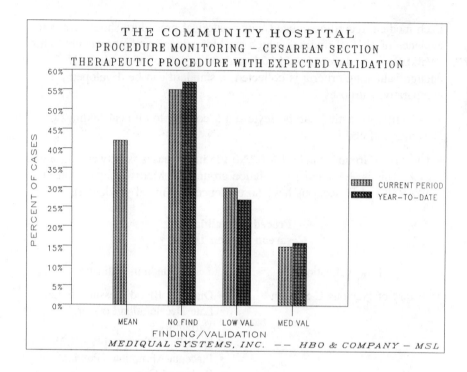

- Community Hospital is higher than the MedisGroups mean for "No Findings" C-Section rate.

- Community may have potential to shift some C-Sections to Normal deliveries. The hospital needs to review C-Section medical records for clinical evidence supporting a high rate of surgical procedures.

Exhibit 8

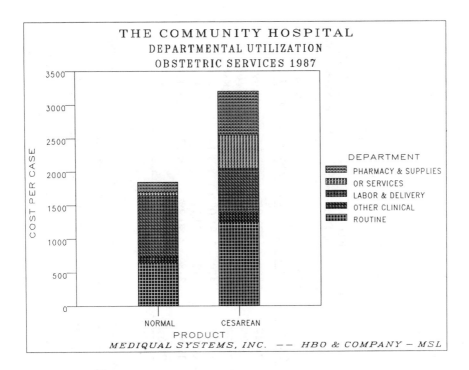

- Utilization for the two primary obstetrics products can be examined by their respective departmental resource consumption.

- A shift in the product mix from C-Sections to Normal deliveries will reduce the average cost per case, some of which can be passed on to PHP as a lower per diem.

Exhibit 9

State Competitive Data Base—Community Hospital
Cesarean Section Profile by Facility

Page: 1
Date/Time: 25-MAR-88, 02:25 PM
CML Data Base: MAOCDB: MADB. CML

	Total Deliveries	Cesarean Deliveries	% Total	Vaginal Deliveries	% Total	Total Del. LOS	Cesarean Del. LOS	Vaginal Del. LOS
Community Hospital	1,115	277	24.8%	838	75.2%	3.04	4.99	2.40
Columbus Hospital	1,767	495	28.0%	1,272	72.0%	3.10	4.16	2.68
Fairview Hospital	1,385	301	21.7%	1,084	78.3%	3.16	4.83	2.65
Parkwood Hospital	591	112	19.0%	479	81.0%	3.14	4.42	2.84
Memorial Hospital	1,904	387	20.3%	1,517	79.7%	3.12	4.15	2.58
St. Mary's Hospital	1,643	325	19.8%	1,318	80.2%	3.17	5.01	2.72
Report total	8,405	1,897	22.6%	6,508	77.4%	3.14	4.53	2.75

- Community Hospital is performing slightly more Cesarean deliveries (24.8%) than the area standard (22.5%). Only through medical record review and action can Community achieve a new utilization pattern of C-Sections.

- Achieving lower utilization of C-Sections will improve quality and lower cost, leading to a competitive advantage.

Exhibit 10

The Community Hospital: Contribution Margin by Product

	Net Revenue	Variable Cost	Contrib. Margin	Cases	Net Rev. per Case	Cont. Mar. per Case
Cesarean Deliveries						
Medicaid	96,884	39,125	57,759	28	3,460.14	2,062.82
Blue Cross	514,245	151,184	363,061	104	4,944.66	3,490.97
Comm. Ins.	312,843	87,234	225,609	62	5,045.85	3,638.85
PHP	198,750	66,408	132,342	53	3,750.00	2,497.02
All Other	117,304	42,829	74,475	30	3,910.13	2,482.50
	1,240,026	386,780	853,246	277	4,476.63	3,080.31
Normal Deliveries						
Medicaid	237,348	104,366	132,982	152	1,561.50	874.88
Blue Cross	579,195	190,036	389,159	265	2,185.64	1,468.52
Comm. Ins.	328,682	101,417	227,265	147	2,235.93	1,546.02
PHP	246,600	99,237	147,363	137	1,800.00	1,075.64
All Other	215,912	83,581	132,331	137	1,576.00	965.92
	1,607,737	578,637	1,029,100	838	1,918.54	1,228.04
Total Deliveries						
Medicaid	334,232	143,491	190,741	180	1,856.84	1,059.67
Blue Cross	1,093,440	341,220	752,220	369	2,963.25	2,038.54
Comm. Ins.	641,525	188,651	452,874	209	3,069.50	2,166.86
PHP	445,350	165,645	279,705	190	2,343.95	1,472.13
All Other	333,216	126,410	206,806	167	1,995.31	1,238.36
	2,847,763	965,417	1,882,346	1,115	2,554.05	1,688.20

- Because Community is operating greatly under capacity, the financial analysis will assume that fixed costs will remain unchanged for the volume levels discussed. Contribution margin will be used as the proxy for profitability.

- PHP experienced 53 Cesarean deliveries at $3,750 per case and 137 Normal deliveries at $1,800 per case during 1987.

- The average cost per case was $2,344 at $750 per day (ALOS = 3.13 days).

- Community Hospital earned $280,000 on PHP's OB business to cover fixed and indirect costs.

Exhibit 11

The Community Hospital: Contribution Margin by Product—Effect of Product
Shift Assuming a 13% Reduction in C-Sections, Shifting Cases to Normal
Delivery

	Net Revenue	Variable Cost	Contrib. Margin	Cases	Net Rev. per Case	Cont. Mar. per Case
Cesarean Deliveries						
Medicaid	83,043	33,536	49,508	24	3,460.14	2,062.82
Blue Cross	445,020	130,832	314,187	90	4,944.66	3,490.97
Comm. Ins.	272,476	75,978	196,498	54	5,045.85	3,638.85
PHP	172,500	57,637	114,863	46	3,750.00	2,497.02
All Other	101,663	37,118	64,545	26	3,910.13	2,482.50
	1,074,703	335,102	739,601	240	4,477.93	3,081.67
Normal Deliveries						
Medicaid	243,594	107,112	136,482	156	1,561.50	874.88
Blue Cross	609,794	200,076	409,718	279	2,185.64	1,468.52
Comm. Ins.	346,569	106,936	239,633	155	2,235.93	1,546.02
PHP	259,200	104,308	154,892	144	1,800.00	1,075.64
All Other	222,216	86,021	136,195	141	1,576.00	965.92
	1,681,373	604,453	1,076,920	875	1,921.57	1,230.77
Total Deliveries						
Medicaid	326,637	140,648	185,989	180	1,814.65	1,033.27
Blue Cross	1,054,814	330,908	723,906	369	2,858.57	1,961.80
Comm. Ins.	619,046	182,914	436,131	209	2,961.94	2,086.75
PHP	431,700	161,945	269,755	190	2,272.11	1,419.77
All Other	323,879	123,140	200,740	167	1,939.40	1,202.03
	2,756,076	939,555	1,816,521	1,115	2,471.82	1,629.17

• Using a "No Findings" rate equal to the MedisGroups mean, some of Community's C-Sections are shifted to Normal deliveries.

• The general reduction in the number of questionable C-Sections has lowered
the number of PHP's C-Sections to 13%.

• This exercise has reduced PHP's average cost per case by $72 from $2,344 to
$2,272.

• The average length of stay declined by 3%.

Exhibit 12

The Community Hospital: Contribution Margin by Product Assuming an Increase to 500 PHP Cases

	Net Revenue	Variable Cost	Contrib. Margin	Cases	Net Rev. per Case	Cont. Mar. per Case
Cesarean Deliveries						
Medicaid	83,043	33,536	49,508	24	3,460.14	2,062.82
Blue Cross	445,020	130,832	314,187	90	4,944.66	3,490.97
Comm. Ins.	272,476	75,978	196,498	54	5,045.85	3,638.85
PHP	367,500	131,563	235,937	105	3,500.00	2,247.02
All Other	101,663	37,118	64,545	26	3,910.13	2,482.50
	1,269,703	409,028	860,675	299	4,246.50	2,878.51
Normal Deliveries						
Medicaid	243,594	107,112	136,482	156	1,561.50	874.88
Blue Cross	609,794	200,076	409,718	279	2,185.64	1,468.52
Comm. Ins.	346,569	106,936	239,633	155	2,235.93	1,546.02
PHP	663,600	286,121	377,479	395	1,680.00	955.64
All Other	222,216	86,021	136,195	141	1,576.00	965.92
	2,085,773	786,267	1,299,506	1,126	1,852.37	1,154.09
Total Deliveries						
Medicaid	326,637	140,648	185,989	180	1,814.65	1,033.27
Blue Cross	1,054,814	330,908	723,906	369	2,858.57	1,961.80
Comm. Ins.	619,046	182,914	436,131	209	2,961.94	2,086.75
PHP	1,031,100	417,684	613,416	500	2,062.20	1,226.83
All Other	323,879	123,140	200,740	167	1,939.40	1,202.03
	3,355,476	1,195,295	2,160,182	1,425	2,354.72	1,515.92

- The product mix shift and reduction in the per diem have been traded off for an increase of 310 PHP obstetric cases.

- PHP's average cost per case has dropped to $2,062–a decline of 12% ($282 per case).

- Community Hospital has earned a contribution margin of $613,000 on PHP's OB business to cover fixed and indirect costs. This change has improved the bottom line by $278,000.

Appendix I
Excerpts from the CompreLink Users' Guide

Send a Message

Getting Started

To get started, you must first pass through two preliminary menus:

- System Main menu
- Communications Network menu.

Follow these three easy steps.

1. If you are at the System Main menu, press the number of the Communications Network option.

2. If you are at another menu, press HOME to get to the System Main menu and then press the number of the Communications Network option.

 NOTE:

You can select a menu option by either typing its corresponding number or by using the arrow keys to move the highlight to your choice and then pressing the ENTER key.

3. From the Communications Network menu, select the "Create/Send Messages" option.

Source: Excerpted from Integrated Medical Systems, Inc., *CompreLink Users' Guide* (Golden, CO: IMS, 1989), with permission.

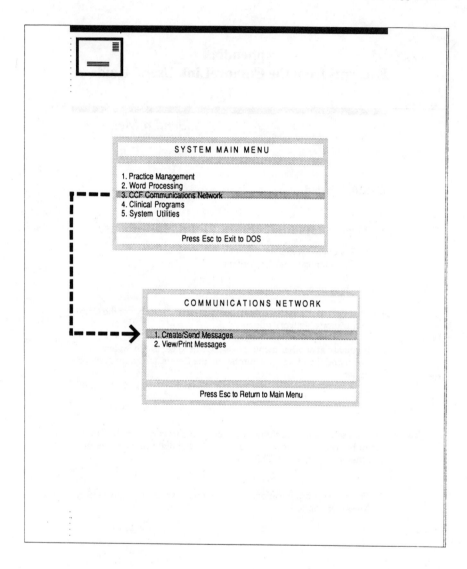

SYSTEM MAIN MENU

1. Practice Management
2. Word Processing
3. CCF Communications Network
4. Clinical Programs
5. System Utilities

Press Esc to Exit to DOS

COMMUNICATIONS NETWORK

1. Create/Send Messages
2. View/Print Messages

Press Esc to Return to Main Menu

Send a Message

Select a Message

Using the CCF Communications Network, you can send five different types of messages:

- *CCF Specialist Appointment* - to request an appointment with a CCF specialist and provide specific patient demographic and diagnostic information

- *Patient Referral* - to refer a patient to any Network participant

- *Diagnostic Results Reporting* - to transmit the results of diagnostic tests to a Network participant

- *General Messages* - to schedule meetings, pose questions to your colleagues or even confirm luncheon arrangements

- *Customized Message Formats* - to call up other pre-formatted message screens that will be developed as needed for your convenience.

To select a message:

1. Select the option for the desired message type from the "Create/ Send Messages" menu.

**CLEVELAND CLINIC FOUNDATION
COMMUNICATIONS NETWORK**

CREATE / SEND MESSAGES

1. CCF Specialist Appointment
2. Patient Referral
3. Diagnostic Results Reporting
4. General Messages
5. Customized Message Formats

Press Esc to Return to Communications Network Menu

YOU HAVE MESSAGES WAITING

HELP   MAIN   Select a function by pressing a number or use the
F1   Home   ↓↑ keys to move the highlight   Select   EXIT
                and then press ENTER   ↵   Esc

Send a Message

Address the Message

The CCF Network message heading acts as an electronic address. It tells the system the name and address of the person/office to which the message is to be delivered.

Addressing the message involves these tasks:

- Write the address (TO and ATTENTION fields)

- Write the return address (FROM field)

- Provide the specifics (ATTENTION and SENT BY fields)

- Specify copies, if desired (COPIES field).

CCF COMMUNICATIONS NETWORK
CREATE and SEND Patient Referral

TO:

ATTENTION:

FROM:

SENT BY:

SUBJECT:

COPIES:

Press ENTER to display network directory.
Enter initials (three CAPITAL letters)
or partial last name of the recipient. Press ENTER

HELP
F1

EXIT
Esc

Send a Message

Write the Text of the Message

Having written the address for the message, you are now ready to write the text of the message itself. The text of your message could:

- Disclose your pre-admission diagnosis

- Specify your admission orders

- Indicate the results of diagnostic tests

- Include any other relevant information.

To write the message text, follow these steps.

1. Use the keyboard to enter information.

2. Make revisions, as desired.

   - Press the arrow keys to move the cursor through the text.

   - Press the BACKSPACE or DELETE keys to remove unwanted characters.

   - Press the INS key to insert additional text.

   - For additional information, press F1 for HELP.

3. Press F10 when finished.

C C F   C O M M U N I C A T I O N S   N E T W O R K
CREATE and SEND Patient Referral

To: Louise Smith MD   Date: 10/16/87   Time: 01:56 PM
 From: Livingston MD, Roger   Sent By: Mary Dunn
Subject: Patient referral for Mr. G.M. Walker
Write the message here:

> I am recommending Mr. G.M. Walker to you for Allergy diagnosis. I
> am attaching my clinical notes on the patient's medical history.

Message Editor: write your message here.
HELP   HOME/END go to start/end of text; PgUp/PgDn scroll the text   DONE   EXIT
 F1   ENTER starts a new paragraph. F10 Completes and exits.   F10   Esc

Send a Message

Finalize the Message

Now that you've written the message, you are ready to finalize it.
From the "Sending Message; Next Action?" menu, you can:

- Print the message on your workstation printer

- Further revise the message

- Save a copy of the message to the disk drive

- Attach a file to the message

NOTE:

The network allows you to attach files to the message you send. For
example, an attached file could contain a patient's medical history or
diagnostic test results. When you send the message you've written, the
system will also automatically send the "attachments" you've included.

The system allows you to:

- View the files you've attached
- Detach a file you've attached
- Send the message.

HOT TIP:

While you complete these actions, the system helps you keep track of
what you're doing. In addition to posting the date and time you created the message, the system also posts the message heading. You'll
find this information just below the Top Message.

C C F   C O M M U N I C A T I O N S   N E T W O R K
CREATE and SEND Patient Referral

To: Louise Smith MD   Date: 10/16/87   Time: 01:56 PM
From: Livingston MD, Roger   Sent By: Mary Dunn
Subject: Patient referral for Mr. G.M. Walker

Sending Message; Next Action?

1. Print this message
2. Add to or review message
3. Save message text to your disk
4. Attach a file to this message
5. View attached files
6. Detach an attached file
7. Send this message

HELP   Select   Select a function by pressing a number or   DONE   EXIT
F1   ↵   use the ↓↑ keys to move the highlight   F10   Esc
                                and then press ENTER.

Index

About the Author

Roger Kropf, Ph.D., is Director of the Health Policy and Management Program in the Wagner School at New York University, where he teaches graduate courses on health care management information systems, strategic planning, and marketing. Previously he was a member of the faculty of the Health Administration Program at the University of Massachusetts at Amherst, where he chaired the university committee on academic computing from 1983 until 1985. He received his Ph.D. from Syracuse University and did his doctoral dissertation on information systems in health maintenance organizations.

Dr. Kropf is the coauthor with Dr. James Greenberg of *Strategic Analysis for Hospital Management,* published by Aspen Publishers in 1984. *Strategic Analysis* describes how information can be collected, analyzed, and presented to support strategic planning in hospitals. Dr. Kropf has published a number of journal articles on strategic planning and information systems and is a member of the Editorial Board of the *Journal of Ambulatory Care Management.* He is a member of the Management Information Systems Task Force of the Association of University Programs in Health Administration and has served as a consultant on information systems to hospitals and state health departments.